MILADY'S GUIDE TO OWNING
AND
OPERATING A NAIL SALON

Delmar Publishers' Online Services

To access Delmar on the World Wide Web, point your browser to:

http://www.delmar.com/delmar.html

To access through Gopher: gopher://gopher.delmar.com

(Delmar Online is part of "thomson.com", an Internet site with information on
more than 30 publishers of the International Thomson Publishing organization.)

For information on our products and services:

email: info@delmar.com

or call 800-347-7707

MILADY'S GUIDE TO OWNING AND OPERATING A NAIL SALON

JOANNE L. WIGGINS

Milady Publishing Company
(A Division of Delmar Publishers Inc.)

NOTICE TO THE READER

Credits:

Publisher:	Catherine Frangie
Assistant Development Editor:	Amy Clinton
Editorial Production:	Laura V. Miller
Production Manager:	John Mickelbank
Art Supervisor:	Susan Mathews
Freelance Project Editor:	Gail Hamrick
Photographer:	Mike Gallitelli on location at Rielms' Hair Studio, Albany, N.Y.

For information address:
Milady Publishing Company
(A Division of Delmar Publishers Inc.)
3 Columbia Circle, Box 12519
Albany, NY 12212-2519

Library of Congress Cataloging-in-Publication Data

Wiggins, Joanne L.
  Milady's guide to owning and operating a nail salon / Joanne L. Wiggins.
    p.   cm.
  Includes index.
  ISBN 1-56253-201-4
  1. Beauty shops—Management. 2. Manicuring.   I. Title.
TT965.W54   1994
646.7'27'068—dc20   93—28026
                                                            CIP
                                                            Rev.

CONTENTS

P R E F A C E

Opening your own salon will in all probability be the greatest
endeavor you will undertake in your business career. Do it right and
it could be the most profitable move you ever make. If you go into
business for any other reason than to be profitable, you will be making
a mistake.

Be prepared to work hard. Watch your expenses and plan, plan,
and plan. This cannot be stressed enough. Start planning your salon
as far in advance of your target opening date as possible. Plan for
every detail. Especially critical is a good business plan. If you need
advice or assistance, seek professional help.

Once you open your salon, practice sound management each
and every day. Analyze your personal management strengths and
needs and work on those areas needing additional development. Set
as one of your goals to be the best manager you can be.

Never stop learning. Stay abreast of the changes in our growing
industry and create the most professional salon in your area. Keep
your staff trained on the latest techniques available at all times. Give
your customers the professional quality services and attention they
cannot get anywhere else. Be the competition; set the standards for
others to try to emulate.

When opening a new salon, the first six months will be the most
critical. Plan on the business interests taking priority over everything

else. Pleasures and other interests will simply have to take second place to your salon and be appreciated later, after your business has become established. As an owner, you must be in the salon and involved in every aspect of your business during this critical period.

Develop your abilities, work hard, and persevere to become a success and achieve all your personal objectives.

Good luck! I know you will succeed.

Joanne L. Wiggins

INTRODUCTION

Would any of us have thought the nail industry (including artificial nails, manicures, pedicures, and nail jewelry) would approach $3.2 billion in income in 1990? Quite frankly, I would never have thought it possible back when I started in the business.

For a quick background, I have been interested in and involved with nails and hand care for my entire adult life. I originally became interested in nails after an operation. While recuperating I began experimenting with artificial nails. I became quite good, at least so my friends told me. Gradually I was persuaded to do their nails out of my home until it simply became too much of an inconvenience. I then found a small commercial space just large enough for a single nail station.

With trepidation I moved in and started my business, just knowing I would embarrass myself to no end. I had never started any kind of business before so this was a bold move for me. After a few months I was so busy and exhausted from the workload and long hours that I was persuaded to hire a technician to help with all the customers. Eventually we were both turning customers away because there simply were not enough hours in the day to handle them and absolutely no room to expand. At that time the only service I offered was sculptured nails and a few manicures. I didn't even sell products.

When a larger commercial space became available in the same complex I moved into it and continued to grow and expand, adding additional services and staff. After a few years, I closed the salon for a complete remodeling. When I reopened, I had a unique salon devoted exclusively to nail care and related services. I was successful beyond my wildest dreams.

When I first started my nail salon there was no information available to help me. Everything I learned was by trial and error. The situation is very different today because the nail industry has grown so much. We now have excellent trade journals, numerous trade shows, and educational schools. We also have products exclusively for the nail industry.

The purpose of this book is to present a concise, semitechnical, authoritative explanation, in easy-to-understand terms, of the principles and practices of salon ownership as based on my personal experiences. I would like to share with you the exciting challenge of taking an idea through all the joys and pitfalls normal to a new venture to a most rewarding future. I would like to share my experiences with you, both good and not so good, so that you may achieve a level of satisfaction and success with as few mistakes as possible.

But first, what kind of person embarks on this type of enterprise? An entrepreneur is defined as a person who organizes and manages a business undertaking, assuming the risk for the sake of profit. However, starting a nail salon involves much more than the above definition entails. An entrepreneur is characterized as having the ability to visualize, to see something that isn't yet created. An "artist" in the business world, this person is usually energetic, optimistic, determined, confident, and single-minded and takes more responsibility for his or her actions than most other people do.

A 1985 study of 468 women entrepreneurs described them as energetic, independent, and goal oriented. They also scored high on competitiveness, self-confidence, flexibility and perfectionism. And what have these entrepreneurs accomplished? Nearly one-third of the small businesses in the United States today belong to women. The number of sole proprietorships owned by women increased by more than 60 percent in the 1980s. From 1980 to 1986, sole proprietorships owned by women rose from 2.5 million to 4.1 million, a 62.5 percent increase. This occurred during a period when the number of male-owned businesses increased 33.4 percent. According to John Naisbitt and Patricia Aburdene in *Megatrends 2000* (New York: Avon Books), the National Association of Women Business Owners (NAWBO) reports, however, that government statistics like these overlook up to two-thirds of women business owners. According to NAWBO, government statistics count only sole proprietorships, probably the smallest firms, not partnerships or corporations. Plus, it says, government figures are three to six years out of date. NAWBO believes that an additional four to five million women business owners have entered the economy in the last fifteen years.

As previously mentioned, it has been estimated that the nail industry alone approached $3.2 billion in 1990, with artificial nails making up approximately one-half of the market followed by manicures, pedicures, and nail jewelry. The nail industry is a woman-dominated industry with 99 percent of the nail technicians being women.

Women's business ownership is obviously the fastest growing segment of entrepreneurship. In 1972, women owned less than 5 percent of American businesses. Today women own approximately one-third of all small businesses. It is estimated that by the year 2000 50 percent of all small businesses in the United States will be owned by women.

Why is this so? Of course there are any number of reasons, but one is that business ownership offers women the opportunity to combine their ambitions with their desire for an active family life. In addition, some women are frustrated with corporate life or feel they have hit the proverbial "glass ceiling"—the level beyond which they no longer can expect promotions.

In these economically difficult times, a nail salon is an ideal business venture because you can start as small or as large as you want. You are limited only by your personal desire, budget, and circumstances.

Nails and nail care treatment is the latest service to be appreciated by the fitness boom. Think about it; your hands are the only part of your body that are always in your line of vision. If your hands and nails look beautiful, you feel beautiful.

Professional nail care service has become a billion dollar industry, and is growing. The average customer spends approximately one-third of her cosmetic budget on nail care. There are certainly tremendous economic opportunities to salon ownership.

When planning to open a salon one of the initial and most important questions you need to ask yourself is whether being a salon owner will improve the quality of your life. Will what you hope to gain with the rewards of ownership and independence be offset or negated by what you stand to lose personally, such as personal relationships or time at home with the family? Successful ownership requires a commitment.

Owning and operating a salon is extremely satisfying—believe me. It's almost impossible to measure. The pride derived from effectively managing a successful salon will usually make all the worry, hard work, and concern ultimately worthwhile. The greatest freedom in life is self-determination, the kind that comes from being in business for yourself.

There are concerns, however, that you and you alone must consider. Can you as a salon owner cope with the decisions and responsibilities of ownership: hiring and firing employees; dealing with unhappy customers; working with landlords, vendors, and employees. If not, then you had best leave ownership and management to someone else. You cannot be what you are not. You need to think through this whole issue of owning and managing a nail salon before you commit yourself, your time, and your resources.

Risk taking is a natural part of all our lives. It causes change and leads to growth. But by clearly thinking through an issue, instead of jumping into it, risks can be substantially minimized. However, once you decide on a course of action, don't look back. Be optimistic. Don't continually be second-guessing yourself. Trust that you made the right decision and move forward with confidence. Plan well, work hard, be appreciative of your success, and have fun being a successful entrepreneur.

There is a tremendous financial opportunity and personal satisfaction to be achieved from salon ownership. But you must be serious, dedicated, and businesslike. Managing a nail salon, or any business, is not a hobby. It is a career.

PREPLANNING

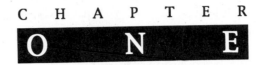

C H A P T E R
O   N   E

My first recommendation is to read through this text completely, from beginning to end, before you do anything. You need to get an overall view of what is involved in owning a nail salon before you even begin to think about what you may or may not want to do. Once you have completed your first reading, start back at the beginning and review the process in chronological order as I have outlined it for you.

TYPES OF SALONS

There are three general categories of nail salons: specialty nail salons that provide specific services only, such as sculptured nails or manicures; full service nail salons that offer a combination of services, such as artificial nails, pedicures, manicures, wraps, and skin care; and service and retail combinations. The very first step is to determine the kind of salon you want to own and manage.

Seek out people who can advise you on the various salon categories. Visit many different salons. What do they do that you like? What do they do that you do not like? Discuss your ideas with family, friends, your attorney, accountant, banker, and anyone else who can give you good sound advice. Before you do anything else, you must know what you want.

MANAGEMENT OVERVIEW

To be successful, profitable, and competitive, and to remain in business over a long period of time, requires sound business knowledge. It requires a basic understanding of management techniques and skills; the ability to control costs and expenses; business development; inventory management; and other areas, such as advertising, customer relations, and personnel relations. Each of these areas and others will be covered later on.

What is meant by management techniques? By effective management? Before you commit yourself and your resources to any business venture you must have an initial understanding of what will be expected of you and of what it will take for you to be successful. Most management texts list five key steps to effective management: planning, organization, delegation, follow-up, and control.

Planning

Planning involves determining the major goals you want to accomplish in one year. It then involves setting goals for two years, three years, and five years. Planning will then involve identifying the intermediate objectives you will have to meet to attain the major goals. To accomplish your intermediate objectives you will need to establish a schedule by working back from a target completion date. You then create a list of all the tasks that must be accomplished to achieve your goal. Arrange the tasks in chronological order. Look at the last task to be completed and determine how much time it will take. Then work back from this target date to establish a start date for the task. Continue this process for all tasks to be scheduled.

Other elements of planning are the establishment of budgets, the identification of required resources and any constraints to your plans, and finally an implementation process.

Organization

Organization involves the setting up of your salon in the style and decor you want, including the actual floor plan. It also involves the selection of employees, development of interviewing guidelines and procedures, creation of a salon policy manual and job descriptions, and determination of salary guidelines.

Delegation

It will be impossible for you to do everything all the time. That's where delegation comes in. Delegation involves letting selected, trusted, and trained employees handle certain responsibilities for you. You will have to choose which functions to delegate, such as inventory control, training, advertising, maintenance, supplies, or educational material. As for each of the key management skills, effective communication with your employees is not only necessary but vital to your ultimate success. It is critical at this stage of your business development. Ineffective communication can make or break your business.

Follow-up

Follow-up is extremely important. A good manager has been defined as a problem preventor and a problem dissolver. Every aspect of your business is ultimately your responsibility. Everything you undertake to establish your business and get it up and running, such as all the planning, procedures, and reports, will be useless if you do not follow-up to confirm that your intentions and instructions have been carried out as you intended. You must be a "hands-on" manager of your employees and your business.

Control

Control is maintaining everything you have worked so hard to build. You must always maintain control of your employees and your salon operating procedures and practices.

If management techniques as briefly presented here are not as developed as you need, review Appendix B for sources of additional information, particularly the Small Business Administration (SBA) resources.

Once you have completed all the preliminary groundwork and decided on the type of salon you want, the next step is to prepare a business plan.

BUSINESS PLAN

What, specifically, are your short-, medium-, and long-term objectives? How will you accomplish these objectives? You need to answer these questions before you go any further. Determine what services (artificial nails, manicures, wraps, pedicures) you want to offer and how much of each service you want to provide. In other words, what will be your mix of services? Do you intend to retail products such as polishes, files, removers, or home maintenance kits? If so, how much and what line? How much of a supply inventory will it take to handle the services you want to provide?

What kind of clientele do you want to attract? This is important because it influences the decor of your salon, the services you offer, and even the type of staff you hire.

You will want to keep your expenses at a minimum, but there will be expenses to accomplish your objectives. You will need to renovate and decorate a chosen location and purchase furniture, equipment, supplies, and inventory. There will be direct and overhead costs such as rent and insurance, and variable costs that vary according to the number and amount of services you provide. You should have a contingency fund for emergencies that should equal at least six months' rent. (Later on, this should be increased to one year.) You will also require sufficient financial backing to sustain you through at least your first year of operation, until income meets and then exceeds expenses.

If you don't know where you are going, fate will take you where it will. With a business plan, you can decide what your salon's future should be and take steps to realize your personal vision. Without a business plan, you are at the mercy of people and events outside your control. Think of a business plan as a road map to get you where you want to go.

Lack of planning leads to crisis management, which takes time and energy away from more productive activities. With a business plan you can define exactly what you want and how you will achieve it, instead of being buffeted by events. You will need to continually grow to survive, and to survive you will need a business plan. Convince yourself you can prepare an effective business plan. It should be simple, practical, and down-to-earth. It doesn't have to be extremely formal, complicated, or drawn out.

Analyze your personal strengths and development needs. Be honest with yourself. Create a personal development plan to work on those areas that must be strengthened. For example, you may be good at planning and customer service but not good with employee training, or you may be good at selecting and providing the services your customers desire but not at scheduling or inventory control. Identify your personal development needs and work to improve them. Once you have satisfied your first plan do the process again and work to improve yet other areas of your personal development.

Establish your objectives and subobjectives for each goal, then develop a series of strategic agendas, backed by practical tactics or action plans, that will allow you to achieve each of your objectives. Establish an implementation process or timetable for completing the various tasks. Finally, create a budget for your plan.

The *USA Today* newspaper published an interview with Joann R. Schultz, a recent winner of the National Small Business Person of the Year, an annual award given by the Small Business Administration. In the award's twenty-seven-year history, Ms Schultz is the first woman to receive it. Her first tip for would-be entrepreneurs is to "prepare a good business plan. If you don't know how, there are books at the library. Have an accountant review the plan. If you can't do a good job, hire a professional. Make sure the plan reflects your goals." I could not have said it better. This is excellent advice.

The Salon

How large (volume of income or number of services) a salon do you want or need? Do you want to create a full-service salon with a large number of employees or do you want a salon with just yourself or perhaps something in between? This in part will be determined by the number of services you plan on providing, the retailing of products, and the image you want to create.

Your salon must have a personality—yours. In my opinion the salon should be excitingly feminine and fashionable, but it must reflect your image. You also have to factor into your considerations what your potential clients expect. They have to feel like they belong, that they are comfortable with the salon image. Your salon personality should complement the type of clientele you wish to attract. In other words, if you were targeting young trendsetters you wouldn't use early American or Victorian decor but probably something very high tech; if you were targeting an older, more affluent, sophisticated clientele you wouldn't go high tech. This is very important. Think it out carefully. Determine the image and personality you want to portray to your clients and even to your employees, and plan accordingly.

Visit other salons for ideas and review trade journals as well as architectural magazines. Look at specific examples of interiors that give you the feel you want to achieve. To a large degree, it is the salon environment, the ambiance, that helps ensure business success. Your salon must look "right" to attract your targeted clientele and even your staff. Know that nail care is a sophisticated, competitive service business. In order for you to be competitive and to continue to remain so, the salon must look the part; it must look successful.

RECEPTION AREA   The reception area is in many ways the most important area in the nail salon. It is the nerve center. It gives your clientele their first (and last) impression of your business—perhaps the most important impression. This area should look comfortable and relaxing with inviting chairs or sofas. It should have attractive accessories, such as retail displays, wall decors, and plants. This area should also include a place to hang coats and hats, preferably close to the entrance.

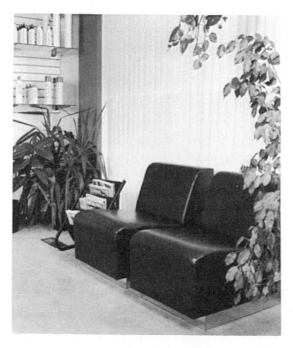

The reception area gives your clientele their first impression of your business.

The reception desk should be large enough for appointment books and telephones and have drawers for incidentals. Also, if possible, there should be a storage area for expensive supplies, confidential information, and retail items. If there is not enough secure desk area valuable items must be locked in another location. The receptionist desk should be situated so that the entire salon can be seen without the receptionist having to get up from the desk. This area should represent approximately 10 percent of the total salon space or up to 20 percent if retailing of products is provided.

Telephones are obviously critical. As a minimum, the receptionist should have two incoming lines for appointments and a separate outgoing line for personal and other calls. The telephones should be located at the receptionist desk for convenience and to discourage use by the staff. Your staff should have a phone for their exclusive use in a break area or in the lunchroom. If your budget will allow it, provide a portable phone for your business clients. Little considerations such as this go a long way to building customer satisfaction.

SERVICE AREA   The service area, or technician working area, will occupy anywhere from 40 to 60 percent of the total salon space depending on the salon image and services offered. The workstations should be uniform, not of mixed furnishings. Proper aisle space between stations is very important to avoid compromising the salon ambiance (and to comply with fire codes and handicap regulations in a public place). It is important to create an image or illusion of space in this area, ideally with the use of primary colors throughout the salon, adding complementary or contrasting shades for accent.

Plan to keep all similar services within common areas, such as nail workstations, pedicures, waxing, facials, etc. Do not mix or intersperse the services throughout the salon.

Pedicures are a rapidly growing service within the nail industry and are often overlooked during the planning and design stage. Pedicure services require additional privacy. I would suggest one pedicure station for every two or three nail stations, preferably located toward the rear of the salon. A built-in sink or foot bath should be part of each pedicure station, again for the privacy of the customers. Pedicure station space should equal approximately 8 percent of the total salon space. Based on the popularity and profitability of this service I strongly recommend you provide pedicures to your clientele.

If other services, such as waxing, skincare, and facials, are a future possibility, try to plan for them during the initial planning stage. These services require even more privacy than pedicures, preferably a separate room. These services could occupy as much as 10 percent of the total salon space.

An alternate guideline for salon size is to allow a minimum of 100 square feet for every workstation. If you have ten stations, you would need a minimum of 1,000 square feet for the salon work areas.

COMMON AREAS   The remaining salon space will be taken up as common areas: 10 percent for walkways and doorways, 4 percent for rest rooms (if not separate); and 6 percent for stock areas and employee lounge or break area.

VENTILATION   Be sure to plan for proper ventilation, i.e., an effective heating and cooling system that pulls air out of the salon while circulating fresh air into the salon. Refer to the Occupational Safety and Health Administration (OSHA) guidelines in order to comply fully with this regulation. Your insurance company should provide loss control service that can assist you with your ventilation requirements and offer suggestions.

LIGHTING   Lighting must conform to your salon image, yet be flexible enough to service an ever-changing assortment of merchandise and displays. Salons require carefully planned, integrated retail displays that depend on being properly lighted. Well-placed lighting and the proper selection of bulbs and fixtures is critical, especially because of the increased number of nail polish shades available in today's fashion-conscious market.

Heavy utilization of incandescent lighting can prove to be expensive. My suggestion is to use a combination of general, accent, and perimeter lighting. When used in moderation, accent lighting provides some relief from the monotony of general lighting. Perimeter lighting is important to make the salon space pleasant, attractive, and comfortable.

Proper lighting can be expensive so get good advice from a lighting specialist, perhaps even several opinions, before you commit your resources. Most large retail lighting establishments have experts who can assist you at no cost. Note, however, that when you are using gels, overhead lights can cure the gel. This is something retail lighting establishments do not know anything about. Check with your product distributor for their suggestions on the effects of various lights.

Location

Your choice of location will be critical. This decision will mean the difference between success or failure. I cannot stress this point strongly enough.

Where should you locate your salon? There are obviously many considerations that must be evaluated:

1. *Competition.* How much competition will you have in any given location? What are their strengths and weaknesses? Do they provide the same services you will be providing?
2. *Walk-in business.* Do you want walk-in customers? The rent will be higher in a high-traffic area such as a mall.
3. *Convenience.* Is the location convenient for the type of customer you plan to attract? How easy will it be for new customers to locate you? How easy will it be for you to give directions to the salon?
4. *Zoning.* What are the zoning and state/city business requirements, if any, among the location possibilities? Check these out very carefully.
5. *Lease option.* If you can't buy a location try for a long-term lease or one with an option to buy. Don't get into a month-to-month rental as you will not be secure about the monthly rental payments increasing. Without the protection of a lease it would also be difficult to build your clientele, justify expenses for adequate decorating, and establish yourself in the area. You must protect your business investment with an adequate lease.
6. *Higher floors.* Don't select a second floor or higher location. Most customers simply do not like higher floor areas. This is also important if you desire walk-in customers.
7. *Shopping Malls.* Avoid shopping malls as the hours are usually restricted. Also, your women customers whose hair may be in curlers will not want to come to your salon if you are in such a public location.

Your local public library, chamber of commerce, and the Census Bureau can provide information on the number of residents, age, income level, family size, and other characteristics of locations you might want to consider. This research will be well worth the time and effort if it prevents you from selecting a location with demographics not in accord with your business plan.

Work with a reputable commercial real estate broker. In addition to helping you select a location, the broker can assist you in negotiating a favorable or at least acceptable lease/rental agreement with better conditions for you. For each location being considered, find out if there are any hidden expenses you will be expected to assume, such as:

Separate water
Other utilities (gas, electricity)
Maintenance
Snow removal or cleanup charges
Association fees

Find out who your neighbor businesses are and if there is the possibility of an unwanted type of business, such as car repair, relocating next to you.

Go slow, be careful, and choose a location you will never regret. Be sure to get everything spelled out and in writing. Have your attorney look over any agreement before you commit yourself and certainly before you sign any contract.

SAFETY AND SECURITY   The safety and security of your clientele, your employees, and yourself is another major consideration. It is your responsibility to protect everyone by providing the first line of protection through the location of your salon. This could also protect you from civil lawsuits involving security negligence.

Give as much thought to the parking area as you do to the interior of the salon. People who intend to rob someone usually prefer areas with shadows and with as little light as possible. Exterior lights should eliminate shadows and dark spots around the salon and in the parking area. Adequate lighting is also important for underground parking areas and in stairways and walkways.

The outdoor parking area should not have any overgrown shrubbery that could provide a hiding place for anyone intent on robbery or vandalism. If there is a fence around the parking lot check for holes and repair them. Always be conscious of safety considerations.

Have any security concerns corrected prior to completing a lease. Specifically, identify and spell out in writing what the lessor (building owner) is to do and by when (ideally prior to your occupancy). Have your attorney explain this to you so you understand it completely before you sign a lease.

Ask potential business neighbors about criminal activity in the area. Check with the local police for any crime activity in the location you are considering. Review the records of an area in approximately a one-mile radius of the location being considered for the last two years. Specifically investigate crimes against people and property. It is your responsibility to evaluate this data. Ignorance will not be a very good defense if you are sued in a court of law.

Do your own personal evaluation of each location, then put yourself in the customers' and employees' position. How will they feel about the location under consideration?

Employee Remuneration

Employee remuneration is also a part of your business plan. The receptionist should be the only employee on a regular salary, which should be based on the local going rate for small business receptionists. If you have your receptionist sell products, pay her a regular salary plus commission to encourage sales. This way the receptionist is a more valuable employee to you who can inform and advise your customers on the various products handled by your salon. Don't pass up any opportunity to make sales.

You may want to pay your technicians a salary while they are in the initial stages of employment and until their work/income reaches a predetermined level. This salary should not be so high that it reduces the incentive of going on full commission. This is also somewhat beneficial as it ensures that new hires won't become discouraged while learning and building up their clientele base. The amount of the commission should be based on experience and how well the technician keeps informed and updated on techniques, how well she interacts with the other employees and clients, and how much she adds to the overall success of the salon. It is quite easy to establish your own criteria for whatever commission levels you choose.

Most technicians are paid anywhere from 40 to 50 percent of their total income to the salon. A relatively inexperienced technician or beginner, starting at 40 percent, should be able to earn 45 percent once she learns new skills with additional techniques, 50 percent with still additional expertise, and even 55 percent if she becomes an extremely valuable employee. However, I would strongly caution you against paying anyone more than 50 percent. You simply will not have enough income left over to cover your expenses and for a satisfactory profit margin.

Duties, training, and responsibilities should all be completely spelled out for each commission level so that there is no misunderstanding on anyone's part. This will help to avoid morale problems and loss of staff that you have invested time, money, and energy to train.

One other remuneration approach is to provide a combination of a base salary plus commission. On several occasions I have used the following: A guaranteed base salary plus one-half of whatever service receipts above the employees doubled salary. For example, suppose you guarantee a base salary of $200 per week. If the employee does $600 of work/income to the salon, the employee would earn $200 plus $100 (one-half of $200 above doubled base of $400) for a total of $300.

Employees should also be paid a commission on product sales, anywhere from 10 to 15 percent, which will encourage sales and increase salon income. This is particularly beneficial if you get into private label product lines.

If you are going to start out small as an owner/operator, plan on hiring your first nail technician when your weekly calendar becomes three-fourths full. As you grow continue to use this simple rule. Do not wait until you are fully booked and turning away customers to hire technicians. You lose business if you do.

I would not recommend that you rent nail stations as you could be liable for their Social Security taxes. Even though you enter into an independent contractors agreement this will not necessarily guarantee your protection.

Budget

Your budget is your financial business plan. It guides your activities toward the most profitable type of business operation and enables you to set goals and identify the steps necessary to achieve them. It is a plan of future receipts and expenditures and a basis on which you can monitor your business activity.

Your first step is to decide what profit you want to make during a given period of time. Then list the expenses you will incur in order to make that preplanned profit. Let's say you want to earn $500 a week in profit. Based on the following assumptions, the salon would have to generate a gross income of $2,500 per week (excluding taxes) to earn this level of income:

Salary/commissions	$ 1,250
Advertising	250
Overhead	250
Supplies	250
Profit	500

Another way of considering the profit issue is to identify as your goal an adequate rate of return for your investment of time and energy plus a return for your financial investment.

You will need to project your fixed costs (insurance, rent, taxes, fixed wages, interest, maintenance, office expenses, and depreciation of equipment) and variable costs (commissions, payroll taxes, insurance, advertising, utilities, supplies). Variable costs vary according to your level of sales/service income.

Establish an annual budget and then break it down into quarters for monitoring purposes. Review your financial budget monthly and adjust your activities if any amount is not developing according to your plan. For example, if the number of customers is ahead of schedule you might want to reduce your advertising. Prepare, or have your accountant do it for you, a quarterly profit and loss statement. You must know how you stand financially at all times. Work with an experienced accountant who understands your business.

BUSINESS NAME

Before we get too far along, let's take care of our egos and get the name of the business out of the way. Be aware that a business name can attract new customers to your salon or discourage customers from entering it. You obviously want to attract new customers. Also, a name can be immediately identifiable with your salon or easily forgotten. When choosing a name for your salon keep in mind the image you are trying to create and one that will reflect your style and spirit.

You will also want the name to identify the services you offer in your salon. The name of your business should be simple, not complicated, but short and catchy.

Avoid common, personal names that could create difficulty if you ever wanted to sell the business, for example names such as "Nails by Rita & John." A new owner would have to assume the business name that he/she might not particularly like or change the name to something else, which would be expensive (signs, advertising, etc.) and could create customer confusion and loss of existing customers. Also, avoid foreign names, initials, and names that may limit your future growth opportunities, such as those that indicate "manicures only."

Conduct a brainstorming session with friends to identify a dozen names then gradually narrow the selection down to one or two. Have your attorney conduct a search for previous or current use of the names you choose to make sure there will not be a legal difficulties with your selection. You should also register the name with the city in which the business is located so they can check the name to avoid any problems.

PITFALLS

You obviously want to avoid as many pitfalls as possible when planning and designing your salon. Avoid impatience that will lead to mistakes that could be very costly later on, both in terms of income and performance results. Once you are completely satisfied that you have considered and planned for every phase of your business development and any issue that may arise, then move forward. Do not attempt to manage without a business and financial plan. Determine what you want to accomplish and plan every detail.

Do not run the risk of running out of money because you failed to view the project in its entirety. Carefully think through everything you want for your salon that involves money. Know what your plan will cost up front, before you start doing anything. If you don't estimate properly, you will run out of money leaving your salon half-finished and not at all what you want. Or your project will simply fail, with you losing your initial investment and possibly even owing additional money. And do not commit all your capital up front. Maintain a contingency fund for the inevitable rough spots.

Remember to budget for adequate advertising needed to attract customers into the salon. Customers are the only source of income to cover expenses.

Also, plan for seasonal cycles, particularly the usually slower summer months when many people are on vacations. The winter months, from November through May, will be your busiest time of the year.

Avoid making changes in your plan while it is progressing. If you planned well you will not need to make changes. Making changes midway can be very costly and disrupt other parts of your plan.

Clear and constant communication with everyone involved with your enterprise is most critical to your eventual success. Only you will suffer if something goes wrong because of a lack of clear communication on your part.

I certainly do not want to give the impression of dwelling on negatives. These points are cautions to be aware of as you proceed through the development of your business plan. On a more positive note, there are keys that will help ensure your success.

KEYS TO SUCCESS

1. Give yourself plenty of time to learn the business. As an owner, you need to be an expert in all phases of salon operations. This is very important. You need to be able to personally train all your employees. If you do not know all the techniques and skills required of each of the services your salon will provide, you will significantly compromise your chance of overall success. You also need to take the time to prepare yourself with management skills in addition to technical skills. Learning technical and management skills is never ending, but be sure you have at least a basic knowledge in both areas.

2. Develop a positive mental attitude. If you are prone to being negative, work on this. Do something to change it. Take whatever steps you need to take to improve and develop a positive mental attitude. Your attitude creates your world. You are what

you think about—good, bad, or indifferent. The individual who says "I can" and the individual who says "I can't" are both correct. You choose which individual you will be. Your business will depend on it.

3. Control your time. This is one of your most important assets and you have only so much of it. Learn to control your time and to schedule it judiciously.

4. Utilize all the resources available to you. You can personally do only so much and you can personally be an expert in just so many areas. You must know your limitations and when to seek professional assistance, such as with nail care techniques, advertising, inventory, or financing There are many sources for assistance, such as the Small Business Administration, trade associations, product manufacturers, community groups and various professionals (bankers, attorneys, insurance agents, accountants). Be sure to check out any and all women's organizations in your area.

5. Be flexible, eager, and willing to accept challenges. The nail industry is not static; it is constantly growing and improving. You must be flexible enough to stay abreast of changes or you will not succeed.

6. Remember that for every problem there is a solution. Don't get discouraged. If you can't resolve the problem yourself, seek outside assistance. The answers or solutions are available. Find them.

7. Decide up front, through extensive study and research, on the exact type of salon you want to create, including the various services you want to offer.

8. Develop a detailed, sound, in-depth business plan. Have your business plan reviewed by someone who can give you an honest, unbiased opinion and assessment of it.

9. Your salon size should be tailored to your business plan. It should not be so large that you are paying for unused space, and it certainly should not be too small.

10. Select a location for your salon that allows you to meet your business plan objectives. Be patient and very selective in choosing your location. Once you sign the papers it will be very difficult (and expensive) to change your mind.

11. Have faith in yourself and in your abilities. Believe that you can compete and be successful. This leads to confidence in yourself that further ensures your success.

12. Be enthusiastic, imaginative, and creative. Visualize yourself being successful even before you start your project or activity. Always strive to have as your personal goal that you will do better than your competitors. Be the best. Set the standards by which others are judged.
13. Develop good people skills. Learn how to work with and understand employees and customers.
14. Provide continuing education for yourself, your technicians, and even for your receptionist.
15. You must have integrity at all times, to be consistent in what you do and say. Always be the best you can, and mean what you say by backing up and guaranteeing your work.

SUMMARY

Give your customers professional, quality services and attention they cannot get anywhere else. Plan on doing the little things that you would appreciate having done for yourself.

Nail care is a wonderful and growing industry, ideal for any individual with an entrepreneurial spirit. The financial and personal rewards can be fantastic, but the key is proper, effective, and in-depth planning. Planning cannot be emphasized enough. If you adequately plan for everything before you commit your time and resources, then your goals and objectives can be achieved.

C H A P T E R
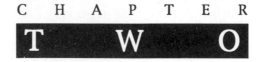
T W O

Before you begin a new business, there are several things that must be done, including obtaining property, which in turn requires investigating and signing a lease, finding a reputable attorney and accountant, and establishing insurance.

Advertising and promotion are critical to your salon's success, especially in the early stages of development when you need to attract new customers. There are many ways to advertise and each is advantageous in its own way.

LEASING A LOCATION

Assuming you are not planning on buying an existing salon or building a salon on your own property, you will need to lease a business location. With your market research and your financial plan completed you are ready to lease a location for your salon. **CAUTION**: Do not sign any lease, or any other type of contract, without first consulting your attorney.

First things first. You must know what you need from the lessor. You need to know what the lessor is willing to provide, then you negotiate. Your best lease option is a one-to-two-year lease with an option to renew for five years at an agreed-upon renewal rate. The

ease should be automatically renewed unless you send notice of
ancellation to the lessor within a time frame specified within the
ease. If you will be subject to rent increases, you need to understand
ιow the increase will be computed. This should be spelled out in very
pecific detail in the lease.

Some other considerations you need to address are:

1. The physical condition of the property. Make sure there are no
   obvious physical problems such as a leaky roof or bad plumbing.
   Also, know whose responsibility it is to repair the problems.
2. Is the location in compliance with local and/or state regulations
   and can you start a nail salon in this particular location? Is the
   building in compliance with existing building codes, zoning
   laws, and regulations?
3. Will the health department and fire department approve the
   operation of your business at this location?
4. How much space are you are leasing? Ideally, you should lease
   net floor space, that is space you will occupy, not areas common
   to other tenants.
5. What will your insurance costs at a particular location be?
   Crime rates as well as location will impact insurance costs. What
   kind of insurance will the lessor require of you? Let your insurance agent review the proposed lease to see if insurance requirements will cost you anything additional.
6. Will there be any restrictions on delivery of merchandise to the
   location?
7. Does the location comply with local regulations regarding rest
   rooms? How many are required? What size? Is sufficient hot
   water available?
8. Are there any limitations or restrictions as regards signage? Will
   you be able to use outdoor signs? What size? Where? How
   often?
9. Is the parking area adequate for customers and employees? Are
   safety concerns satisfied? If not, can they be made satisfactory
   and who will do what, by when? Who will pay?
10. Is the electrical power sufficient with enough outlets for your
    planned stations and reception area? If not, what will be the cost
    to bring the premises up to minimum standards and who will
    pay? Watch out for utility-sharing agreements and energy escala-
    tion clauses. These could become expensive for you.

11. Is the climate control (heating/air conditioning) adequate for your planned operation? Is the ventilation adequate? You will need more ventilation if you plan on doing a significant amount of acrylic work.

12. Who has the responsibility of maintenance/repair? This should be the lessor. Avoid a lease that allows the lessor to repair the premises at your expense.

13. Can you guard against undue competition by including a statement restricting the lessor from leasing other locations to businesses similar to yours?

14. Will you be able to sublet the premises if you have to? What would be the conditions/restrictions? This could be important if you have to move your business before your lease expires or if you want to rent station/floor space to outside technicians.

15. What happens to improvements you make to the premises? Can you get a credit for the expenses or take the improvements with you?

16. How can you get out of the lease? Know the penalties (if any) as well as time frames.

17. How much security deposit is required? How and when do you get it back? Get very specific and don't have any misunderstandings. Will your deposit earn interest and will it be credited to you? It should.

Review everything with your attorney. Know what you are getting and know all of the financial specifics, in detail. Be sure you know how you can get out of the lease and what it will cost you. And remember to put everything in writing—**everything**.

PROFESSIONAL SERVICES

The best advice I can give you about any service that is not your personal specialty is to seek professional advice and assistance. Your attorney and accountant can aid you in obtaining the necessary operating licenses and permits and help you register with the appropriate government agencies. They can also counsel you in obtaining needed financing.

In advance of opening your salon, you have to submit the necessary applications with the state and local government agencies to get the required business forms and tax permits. Before you can legally open your business, you must have obtained all of your proofs of permits and each must be in your possession, in force, on site, and clearly posted. This of course includes your personal licenses (manicures license, beauty school certificate, or whatever type of specific training your particular state requires).

Be sure you understand:

- The various business ownership structures, such as sole proprietorships, partnerships, and corporations.
- Tax considerations, such as investment tax credits; subchapter "S" treatment for corporate accelerated depreciation; and tax reporting of sales, income, Social Security, and employee/employer taxes.
- The difference between employees and independent contractors.
- Accounting methods: cash, accrual, etc.
- Employee taxes and record keeping, group insurance plans, workers' compensation insurance, federal and state unemployment insurance.
- OSHA requirements.
- Retirement plans.
- Insurance—general liability and product liability, premises/contents, malpractice, fire, business interruption, and workers' compensation.

Your Attorney

If you don't already have a trusted attorney, finding the right one for your business will require planning and research. Put together an inventory of your needs. Try to find someone who has already demonstrated expertise in your field.

You can speak to other business owners in your area, or ask other professionals, such as your banker, accountant, or insurance agent for references. Lawyer referral services are of questionable value since some charge a fee to attorneys to be listed and most do not discriminate as to who they list. Local bar associations are also of questionable value because most referrals are for less experienced attorneys and most do not categorize their members by specialties.

You want an attorney with whom you have a good chemistry, someone who will have time for you when you need it, who will be available, and who has the experience you need.

Once you have chosen an attorney, but before you actually meet him or her, you will want to check credentials and abilities. Verify with the bar association that the attorney is licensed in your state and whether any disciplinary actions have ever been taken.

During your initial visit with your prospective attorney you must discuss and understand the attorney fee schedule. Ask questions. The most common method will be an hourly fee schedule. Find out if the attorney has a minimum fee per transaction, for example if you call the attorney and talk for one minute, will you be charged for thirty minutes or for a minimum amount of time? Also check out contingency fees and retainers.

Once you choose an attorney, as a minimum you should expect him or her to review any existing contracts, leases, insurance policies, and, if incorporated, your corporate records and offer any pertinent advice.

Don't wait for a crisis to select an attorney when time becomes a critical factor and your choices may be limited. Adequate legal planning and preparation can often result in a crisis being averted entirely.

Consider your attorney as part of your business team, with you as the captain. Remember, to establish a good attorney/client relationship you must be honest at all times and keep your attorney informed of any changing facts related to your business. Also, write to your attorney when convenient instead of always calling on the telephone, and don't expect an attorney to work without being paid.

Your Accountant

To be successful, you must also achieve effective financial management. This means that an accountant can be most helpful to you.

You must establish records of cash receipts, cash disbursements, sales, purchases, payroll, equipment, inventory, accounts receivable, and accounts payable. You can either keep this information yourself, hire someone else to keep it, or pay your accountant to keep it.

In addition to preparing and analyzing your profit and loss statement and helping you identify areas that need financial control, an accountant can give you advice on financial management, cash management, budgeting, forecasting, borrowing, benefits of various types of business organizations (sole proprietorships, corporations, etc.), and taxes. Again, consider your accountant as part of your business team.

As with your attorney, you will need to check on the qualifications and the integrity of your accountant. Get references and check them out carefully. Be selective. As with anything, the cheapest or lowest cost is not necessarily the best bargain in the long run.

Your Insurance Agent

If you want to be in business you must have insurance. Accept this fact and shop around for your best buy. You would not believe the potential for large financial loss from the operation of a business in today's legal environment. With insurance, what you are in effect doing is substituting a relatively small loss (the insurance premium you pay) to buy protection against a potentially very large or catastrophic loss. Not only is insurance necessary and a smart business investment, some insurance is required by law in most states (workers' compensation and/or automobile).

Your insurance agent should be able as a minimum to explain malpractice insurance, automobile insurance, products liability, fire, workers' compensation, premises liability, and life/medical insurance. Your agent should work with you to identify and evaluate your potential exposures to various losses, how much liability you could assume, the amount and type of deductibles, and what amount of insurance to buy and from which insurance company.

As with the other members of your business team, select your insurance agent carefully. Select an agent who comes well recommended and who has been in business successfully for a long time.

There are basically two types of insurance agents: those who are employees of "direct-writers" and sell insurance for their employer only, and agents who are independent businesses such as yourself and represent one, two, or any number of different insurance companies. Personally, I would recommend that you secure as many quotes from as many different agents as you feel necessary. The insurance industry is very competitive so shop around for the best price and service for whatever insurance coverage you need.

Also, if possible, try to get all your insurance coverages from one agent and from the same insurance company. If you ever have a claim this could be of benefit to you. This may not be practical but at least try. As a prudent businessperson, it is your decision and ultimate responsibility to make sure you have adequate insurance protection and that your insurance program is reviewed and updated regularly, particularly as your business grows and your needs change. Remember, you are insuring your business dream, so make sure your insurance agent appreciates your protection needs.

ADVERTISING AND PROMOTION

There are two kinds of advertising: that which is effective and that which is not. The second kind is never worth the cost, whatever the cost may be. The first kind is always worth the cost. Regardless of what has been spent and what has been saved, the financial bottom line of your business is the important consideration. Effective advertising and promotion is critical to your salon success, especially in the early stages of your business development until you have more customers than you can service. A good beginning rule is to spend 10 percent of your gross monthly income on advertising. You would then adjust your advertising expenditures up or down as your business matures.

There are many ways to advertise:

Outdoor signs	Magazines
Telephone books	Trade publications
Print ad coupons	Trade associations
Newspaper display ads	Direct mail
Television	Handouts/promotions
Shopping guides	Radio
In-house customer incentives	Referrals

The best and most effective is word-of-mouth customer referrals achieved through superior, quality service to your existing clientele.

The main reasons customers choose to frequent one salon over another are:

1. Quality of service.
2. The way you make them feel, not just look.
3. Cleanliness.
4. Location.
5. Hours of operation.

You will want to highlight these points in whatever advertising/ promotion vehicles you choose.

Customer referrals are the most impressive and effective advertising of all. They are the least expensive and the most creditable. New businesses obviously cannot rely solely on referrals but must resort to effective media advertising to build a customer base. But don't ever underestimate the value and cost effectiveness of referrals. Ideally, all your business should come from customer referrals.

Costs

How much should you spend on advertising? As much as you can afford to spend. The more the better in order to get your business established. But spend carefully and only on the forms of advertising that will justify the expense.

You will need to identify your advertising objective. What do you want to accomplish with your advertising message? To attract new customers, maximize client retention, build or maintain your community image, or sell slow-moving inventory? You must identify your advertising objective before you spend your dollars, develop your message, and schedule your program.

You might establish a fixed amount for spending on advertising based on what you feel you would need in order to accomplish your business plan objective. A second alternative is to spend a certain percentage of income on advertising. There are no hard and fast rules or methods for determining your advertising budget. However, most salons do spend between 2 and 10 percent of their gross monthly income on advertising.

Avoid spending too little on advertising, which is a common mistake with salons just starting out. Budget and spend a sufficient amount to be effective. Half-hearted attempts will be ineffective, discouraging, and wasteful.

There are two factors that determine the success or failure of any advertising program: the media you choose and the content of your message. Choose your media carefully and work on the message you want to deliver.

Print Advertising

Print advertising, if utilized in a major way, can be expensive. Unless you have experience, for your first effort I would strongly advise you to hire a copywriter to assist you. Afterwards, with the information gathered and knowledge gained, you will be better able to write your own advertising copy.

A good beginning would be to make a list of all the relevant factors about your business that you might want to use in your advertising. Then prioritize your list by how important these factors would be for your target customers. Be sure to rely on careful research to identify which factors are really important to your customers instead of relying on your personal feelings or thoughts. This becomes the theme for your advertising. You are responding to your clients' needs, letting them know that you have what they want.

Develop a realistic and attention getting headline. You will want to stress benefits for the customer instead of features of your salon. Most people are more interested in results than reasons. Always consider your advertising from the customers' perspective. Appeal to their interests. Give them a reason for wanting to come to your salon. Stress only one or two key benefits in each advertising message. Trying to stress too many benefits becomes counterproductive.

Newspapers, mailers, magazines, flyers, and the telephone Yellow Pages are all examples of print advertising you can utilize.

The best way to measure the effectiveness of print advertising is with the use of coupons. Some people suggest putting an expiration date on coupons to give the impression that the offer is limited and should be acted upon within the time frame indicated. However, when first starting out, I feel that you should not use an expiration date because you want new customers any time you can get them with no restrictions.

When using coupons, if the media has editions for different geographical regions, you will need to put a code on the coupons to monitor the effectiveness of the advertising in the various regions, for example N for North edition, W for West edition, etc. This way you can monitor the results more effectively.

For print advertising you might want to explore the use of "gang runs." Large printers often print big runs all at one time, and will fill in with small, unscheduled jobs. Talk to your printer and let them know that you would wait awhile if they would discount your advertising job. Some printers charge one-fifth the normal rate under these circumstances.

Placement of print advertising is important. The upper right-hand side of the page is the best eye-catching spot for your message.

Radio

Radio advertising is usually practical and cost effective for a nail salon. However, this medium may not be particularly good for your specific advertising goals and objectives. You will have to evaluate the potential benefit very carefully. You will have to determine what you expect the advertising to do for you. A single-location salon in a large radio market with limited staff probably will not be able to handle the business resulting from a successful and effective radio advertising campaign. However, a multilocation salon business might very well find radio advertising to be cost effective. However, if you are changing locations or just beginning to build your clientele, radio could be ideal for any size salon.

Targeting your advertising is important. Radio is a direct or "rifled" advertising approach (as opposed to television) aimed at sending a message to a narrow demographic listening audience. Radio is specialized and segmented, with individual radio stations appealing to a specific demographic profile, such as age group, income level, and other personal statistics of the prime listening audience for that particular radio station marketplace. Radio station formats are varied: news/talk, music, or any combination, with music type ranging from country to classical. Each radio station has its own primary listening audience that may be ideal or totally inappropriate for your target market.

Then you have AM or FM radio. Most adults prefer to listen to FM and are often loyal to their particular station. Also, FM stations usually appeal to a narrower range of audiences, which makes it easier to target your advertising efforts. AM radio stations do have their benefits though, so you need to check out your local situation.

Advertising costs will vary from station to station and from market to market. Every station has something similar to a marketing department that can discuss their particular demographic details and advertising rates. They will usually have more data than you will need in order to do your own analysis. You will also find most of them very cooperative in working with you on the kind of advertising that fits your budget.

In addition to reviewing the individual station demographics to determine which radio station to consider, do an analysis of which stations your customers listen to. When do they listen to the radio the most? What time of day? What station do you listen to in the salon?

In the car? Do a study to give yourself better information with which to make a decision.

With radio it is critical that you select the right voice to give your message. Radio provides the sound while the listener develops a mental picture from the advertising words (your message). Interview and keep looking until you find the "right" voice. The radio station will help you identify the right person for your salon. Then use the same voice consistently, just as you would use a business logo consistently.

The content of your radio message should be short and simple. Target your message for the ear. Use action words to sell benefits and solutions. Use short words and sentences to get right to the point of your message. Tell your message in a personal manner; think of "sharing" information with the radio listening audience.

Humor, if done well, can be very effective in this medium. However, humor that fails can be a disaster so be very careful. Humor that is successful is really tough to achieve, but worthwhile if it works for you.

Avoid unrealistic and unbelievable hype. It just doesn't work with today's sophisticated customers. Also, avoid technical or trade jargon in all your advertising. Be conversational in tone and use language that everyone can understand.

You will want your message to get your audience's attention within the first seven to ten seconds. Then your message should inform your listener and finally reward them for listening. After the recording of your advertising message has been completed, personally review it to make sure it meets your requirements. You might even want to attend the recording sessions; you'll find this experience interesting.

Review your message for clarity, believability, and persuasiveness. For a sixty-second radio commercial make sure your salon name and telephone number is mentioned at least three to five times. Finally, make sure you haven't left out the obvious—your salon location.

Television

Television is a "shotgun" approach to advertising that is, in my opinion, not well suited for a nail salon. The viewing audience is just too broad to be cost effective. Television advertising is too expensive for a nail salon to justify unless it is for a large chain of salons within a relatively large area. However, if you do television advertising, make arrangements to get the top newspeople into your salon for complementary services. Give them the works. Once they experience your services their enthusiasm for your advertising will be even higher. This is particularly beneficial if the announcer for your advertising is a woman. Also, since television newspeople are celebrities in themselves, it's good for your other salon customers, i.e., to be a customer of the same salon as "Jane TV Person."

Telephone Yellow Pages

Telephone Yellow Pages have an incredibly high usage among the general public. Fully 97 percent of the public use the Yellow Pages regularly. Although businesses in general are starting to complain about the increased number of telephone directories in use, the public finds them useful. Many say they use two or three different Yellow Pages regularly. I do.

Because there are so many different Yellow Pages printed, you will need to identify which ones are most useful for your particular clientele and target market. Once you decide where your customers come from, and where new customers might come from, your choices will be fewer and easier to make.

Next, you will have to consider which specific headings to use. Consider where your customers would look first. You will probably want to be listed under several different headings, such as manicuring, beauty salons, and artificial nails, in order to attract more customers. The Yellow Pages representative will work with you to help determine the best approach for you to take. You may want to have just single line entries (name and telephone number) versus a display ad. Of course your budget will decide part of this for you as display advertising costs much more than single-line advertising. Remember, advertising in the Yellow Pages is on an annual basis and you cannot change your ad once it is listed.

Be sure to track the results of your Yellow Page advertising. Ask your new clients which directory they used to find you, which heading they looked under, what specifically caught their attention so that they called you. You will then use this information next year when you again start planning your advertising message.

Yellow Page advertising does work. Your message is in front of readers who are in the mood to buy or who are specifically looking for services you and your competitors are offering. For a new salon, your advertising message puts you in the same league as all other salons, no matter how large they are or how long they may have been in business. You have as good a chance of attracting a new customer as any other salon.

If you decide on a display ad be careful of the costs, which can get out of control. It takes many, many new customers a month to justify and cover a monthly expense that can run into the hundreds of dollars. However, if you do use display advertising, make it factual, specific, and believable. Give readers the information they need and include as much as you can in the space you have. What is omitted from your ad can be interpreted as not existing. Include your hours of operation, services, and anything special or unique about your salon. And use your salon logo and graphics to improve the impact of your message.

Because Yellow Pages only come out once a year, call as soon as you can to find out the next deadline. If you miss it by a day, you miss it by a year.

Direct Mail

Direct mail is another useful and beneficial means of getting your message out to your target customer base. Direct mail efforts can be as simple as a post card or can be extremely complex.

The major advantage of direct mail is that you can be selective and make your direct mail as specific or as broad as you wish, depending on your budget, your target market, and your demographics. You have complete control over the scheduling and costs. Direct mail is also the best and easiest of all forms of advertising in which to monitor and evaluate the results of your message.

If you are just starting out in business you will not have your own mailing lists. However, lists are available from list brokers or list houses, such as the telephone company and various organizations. As your business grows and you become more developed you will have your own lists from which to work.

With direct mail advertising limit your message to only one service or product. Don't try to overwhelm the reader. Remember what gets your attention when you receive a mailing and learn from other people's mistakes. For your mailings, two colors are usually better than one. As for the quality of the paper, use only the minimum level of quality necessary. Watch your costs.

Newsletters

A salon newsletter generates tremendous visibility and interest for a salon, perhaps more than any other media vehicle. A newsletter is really a must to round out a successful advertising program. The combination of product and service, education, information, news, special and unique services/benefits your salon offers makes a newsletter an unlimited advertising, promotion, and public relations vehicle. It helps to establish professionalism and a high profile and improves your creditability with your customers. It will help to retain your clients and it will improve your opportunity to increase your goodwill with all of your customers. It will also improve staff morale. A salon newsletter can be used to:

- Explain the benefits of your services, such as manicures, waxing, pedicures, and/or facials.
- Announce changes to your salon procedures or policies.
- Introduce new products or services.
- Introduce new employees.
- Announce product or service promotions and limited-time offers.
- Provide helpful advice or hints for home maintenance of nails, such as how to use a file, the kind of polish to use, or how to use a pencil to dial a telephone.
- Give salon history.
- Generate interest in products and services.
- Make various announcements, such as staff promotions or birthdays.
- Suggest gift ideas your customers can use.
- Announce the latest trends in polish color, nail care, or fashions.
- Feature articles by employees or even customers.
- Announce special community service or charity functions that involve the salon, employees, or customers.
- Provide an information outlet for anything else you can think of that fits your customers' needs, such as recipes and miscellaneous announcements.

Local libraries usually have an excellent selection of books on newsletter production.

You will want to avoid certain topics in your newsletter such as gossip, criticisms, or comments about other salons. The last thing you want is a libel claim or to appear unprofessional.

Costs will vary depending on the length of your newsletter, the quality of the paper used, frequency of publication, and the methods of distribution. Your costs will be quite different if you use it as a handout in your salon rather than mailing it. If you decide to mail the newsletter check with the post office for a bulk-mail permit that can save you a significant amount of money. There are restrictions with these permits, however, so get the details and fully understand what you can and cannot do.

Publicity

Publicity is an element of advertising and promotion that costs relatively little but achieves excellent results. Publicity is free and quite believable, improves creditability, and establishes you as an authority in your field. The only drawback, unlike your own advertising, is that you cannot control when the publicity material or information will be published or in exactly what form. All of this is in someone else's hands, either the editor or media person.

Your first steps in getting free publicity are to identify your market and where your customers are; decide which media is best for your location and needs; and determine what is newsworthy, interesting, and unique about your salon, products, and services. You must understand that editors publish material and stories that appeal to their readers. By understanding their audience you can craft your material to their interests. You have to identify the media's particular "angle" and appeal to it.

Your next step is preparing your presentation. The publicity or press release is in the form of "news" about your salon, such as introducing something special or unique, an expansion, a new product or service, a community donation or service, or free demonstrations. Your story/presentation may be printed as you wrote it or it may be edited by the media. There are general acceptable rules to follow when submitting your write-up:

1. Put the date in the upper right-hand corner.
2. Put the name and telephone number of the person the media can contact if they need to under the date.

3. Put a requested release date under the contact name, either a specific date or "immediate."
4. Prepare a headline for the article.
5. Type, using wide margins and double-spacing, on 8 1/2-by-11-inch white paper. Start the wording approximately one-third down from the top of the paper.
6. When using additional pages, put the headline on the top left-hand corner of the second and subsequent pages.
7. Prepare your write-up in clear, short sentences. Do not use personal opinions or unnecessary adjectives.
8. At the end of the article, centered below the last line, type a symbol such as "#######" or "******" to indicate the end.
9. Send the write-up to the attention of a specific individual or to the editor. It is best to call and ask for the name of the person responsible for receiving publicity releases. Include a short note introducing yourself and the reason for the release.

Most editors suggest using the "inverted pyramid" style of writing for a release. This technique requires that you put as much of the important information as possible at the beginning of the article with lesser facts and information toward the end. This technique allows the reader to get the critical information without reading the whole article or allows the editor to edit from the bottom up if there are space restrictions. The first paragraph is the most critical part of any release. Work on this to make sure it is just right. Concentrate on what the article is about, where it is, who it is about, and when it is.

You can send photographs if you want to and if they add to your article. Use professionally prepared (no *Polaroid*™ pictures or snapshots) photographs, black and white, 5" X 7" or 8" X 10". On the back of each, attach a note with the name of the article to which it applies. Always identify any individuals in the photograph by name and position.

Always call the media you are interested in using to find out about deadlines. Within a few days of sending your release, call to verify that the article was received; do not ask if or when the article may be used. Be satisfied that it will be considered. You will be surprised at how often publicity releases are used by your local media.

When trying to use free publicity, send articles or materials as often as you think they are newsworthy. Also, send your information to more than one publication.

If your article is printed, make copies to use as handouts and as part of your direct mailing effort. Also, frame a copy to use in your salon. This will be very beneficial for your creditability.

Community Involvement

As a salon owner you will be contacted repeatedly to work on various community service activities. But you will also find that the time and service effort required to establish your business will preclude time for active involvement. The time you have available during the initial building stages of your business is finite so you must use it judiciously.

Instead of a personal time commitment, however, many community activities involve auctions or sales programs to generate income for their causes. For charitable activities, a donation of a gift certificate for services is a wonderful way to contribute and at the same time receive good exposure within the community. Until such time as you can afford to commit your time this would be a good alternative.

Once you find yourself free enough to become involved in community services, you will find the effort rewarding on a personal and business level. Your involvement certainly will be beneficial from a publicity standpoint. You might consider offering your services at a local fund-raising event and donating your proceeds to the sponsoring organization. You might volunteer your services to a retirement home or by providing beauty seminars at monthly meetings of various women's organizations. The more community service events you participate in, the more free publicity you will receive.

If community service organizations are not calling you, call them. Tell them that as a community-minded person you want to give something back to your community by offering your services.

Once you become involved with a community event you need to take the initiative to make sure your involvement is recognized. In your local area identify the editors and producers of women's interest programs. After the event, send a press release to everyone on your list, giving the "who, where, what, when, and why" type of information. Within a few days, personally follow-up with the editor to make sure your press release was received and to ask if they need any additional information.

Telemarketing

Telemarketing is simply marketing over the telephone. It is relatively inexpensive and if the sales message is thought out thoroughly beforehand, and if the calls are handled professionally, might be effective. However, I really do not think this is time or cost effective for a nail salon. But if you do try it, I would suggest you consult with a professional firm specializing in telemarketing before you start. They would be able to assist you with acquiring qualified lists of telephone numbers to use.

Outdoor

The use and success of billboard and/or poster advertising campaigns depends upon the placement of the billboard or poster. For them to be effective there must be high traffic count in areas you want to target. Posters can be inexpensive and successful, particularly if placed in locations frequented by your target clientele.

Promotions

Well-thought-out and planned promotions are a vital element in the all-around operation of a successful salon in today's marketplace. As with advertising in general, promotions should be targeted to specific objectives, and to reinforce or build upon your reputation as being the salon to visit for professional nail care. Promotions take many forms:

- Direct mailings at least semiannually to current and inactive customers.
- A customer newsletter, either your own or one subscribed to through a newsletter service.
- Print advertising media.
- Announcements through mailing lists, radio spots, small newspaper ads, or flyers.
- Specially designed salon days, such as Grandmother's Day, Teens-Only Day, Brides-to-Be Day, Secretaries' Day, Men's Night, or whatever "Day" you can think of that will attract a new group of customers to your salon.

Promotional material, such as having your business name, address, and telephone number on pens, pencils, matchbooks, or coffee mugs, is usually inexpensive. However, this type of promotion is often ineffective for bringing in new customers. This type of promotional material is, however, ideal for use with seminars or demonstrations as promotional tools or as gifts.

Be sure to have a large supply of quality, distinctive business cards that you can pass out freely. Include the name of your salon, your logo, your services, hours of operation, address, and telephone number.

Important Reminders

- Advertising and promotions are intended to build your salon business and your standing and image in the community.
- Know what your target market wants and direct your advertising and promotions to those wants.
- Always stress service over price because this is what customers really want.
- In addition to other means, do your research on the working floor of your salon, making everything else secondary to serving the customer.
- Success depends on your commitment to gathering relevant marketing information on a regular basis.
- Periodically reassess your market niche, to identify and evaluate needed changes.
- Don't rely on price alone to attract and retain customers as this creates an impression of downplaying quality and your expert services. Customers will perceive you as a purely price salon.
- Don't overspend or commit to a contract requiring a certain or fixed amount of advertising.
- Keep ads small. A thirty-second broadcast commercial accomplishes almost as much as a sixty-second spot, for less money. The same is true with print advertising. Consistency of advertising is much more important than size.
- Negotiate for media time. Broadcasters have a fear of unsold advertising time. Many would rather settle for a discounted price than waste a spot entirely.
- Stay consistent with your advertising. Run the same ad until it stops working for you. Don't change too frequently.

DECOR

Always keep in mind that your customers are coming to your salon as a treat to themselves. They want to be cared for and pampered. Your customers must be comfortable or they will go somewhere else with their business. You must decorate to appeal to the majority of your potential clientele, not to satisfy your own personal likes and/or whims.

First, remember that you cannot do all the decorating yourself. Second, know your customers and yourself. You want to create an image; know what it is. I would offer that the image should be one that is open and uncluttered with an airy feeling, yet one that provides a sense of privacy. There are many images you can create, but you have to identify what it is you want up front, before you do anything else. Do you want an image that is casual and informal, fast-paced and energetic, businesslike, crazy and fun, chic and sophisticated, or something else?

Don't make any decisions concerning what you will put in your salon until you have completely analyzed your customer, your location, your goals for the salon, and everything else you plan to do for the interior and exterior. Otherwise, you make a mistake.

Eighty to eighty-five percent of your decorating budget will be spent on big basics, such as carpeting or floor tiles, wall coverings, furniture, and lighting. The remainder will be spent on the finishing touches.

Working with a budget means you will not have unlimited funds available for decorating. Therefore, take care of the essentials first. Find out if you need a permit for the kind of ventilation system you want to use, or to install electric fixtures or plumbing. Is a rest room required and if so how large? Find out if a special rest room with facilities for the handicapped is required. Rest rooms should be as large as possible to allow the customer to change clothes prior to pedicures. They should also have well-lit mirrors and coat hangers or hooks.

Before you start, make a "wish list" of everything you want or would like to have in your salon, then balance your ideal decorated salon with your budget. Be sure to take into consideration all of the services you want to offer and the number of stations for each service. Consider all services, including the reception area and retail area. Be sure to anticipate and plan for adequate plumbing and electrical installations.

Your local furniture distributors are usually a good source of advice when it comes to decorating. Also, your local university or college may have interior design departments and would appreciate the opportunity to work with you for the experience. Check out every possibility for advice and ideas.

Color

Color of course is an extremely important consideration when decorating. Start with the major or dominant wall areas and floors, then go on to the secondary areas (windows, large pieces of furniture), then choose accent colors for the accessory pieces. Don't choose a color just because it is fashionable. Choose one for your customers, employees, and yourself.

You should know that different colors can excite, stimulate, relax, depress or even tranquilize different people. Colors even affect people who are color impaired! Color can affect not only moods but physical well-being. You will want to select colors for your clientele, not what you personally like or dislike. However, note that reactions to color are so varied that it is impossible to decorate to please everyone all the time. Also, some people's reactions to color are associated with their culture, nature, language and personal experiences. The best you can do is to appeal to the majority of your clientele.

When selecting colors I recommend that you use shades and tints, as opposed to primary colors (red, blue, yellow) that will result in color schemes that please a majority of the people. Once you understand basic color principles and how color will affect the salon, you can begin to choose your color scheme. For example, red can be exciting, bold, and stimulating yet is considered by some to be aggressive and overpowering. Blue can be considered calming, cool, and relaxing yet is considered by some to be sad, depressing, or draining. The examples go on and on. See the color chart, page 43 for additional information.

Flooring and Carpeting

When it comes to flooring, be as careful and accurate with your floor measurements as possible. Costs can add up quickly. If you use carpet you will need a commercial grade not a residential grade. Be sure to get warranties on all material and workmanship.

Fabrics

For fabrics, check to see if there are any local board of health codes regarding fabrics in your area. When purchasing fabrics, don't buy on price alone. Consider what you need as regards the heat, sun, light, and cold in addition to the esthetic appeal. Also, consider fire retardant qualities and ease or difficulty of cleaning.

COLOR

PRIMARY COLORS: Red, blue, and yellow.
SECONDARY COLORS: Green, orange, and purple.
> Result of mixing two primary colors, i.e., yellow plus blue equals green.

VALUE of a color refers to the lightness or darkness of a color and can be changed by
> adding white or black. Value is what gives an object shape and puts perspective and depth to the work.
> > Adding white gives a tint.
> > Adding black gives a shade.
> > Adding black and white gives the tone.

WHITE is the absence of color.
BLACK is the presence of color.
When mixing, always start with the light color and add the darker color to it to create the
> effect you want:
> > Yellow + black = dark forest green
> > Yellow + blue = spring or moss green
> > Yellow + red = orange
> > White + red = pink
> > Red + blue = purple

Examples of color impacts:
> Red/yellow: Can raise blood pressure and pulse rates, indicative of being jumpy, nervous, risk taking, active, bold.
> Blue/pink: Calm, relaxing, soothing.
> Shades of orange, red, yellow: Can stimulate appetite.
> Pink: Very feminine. May turn men off.
> Black/white: Wealth and power. Says we provide the background, you set your own style.
> Neutral beige, taupe, and light grey: Calming, soothing and relaxing.

Blue:	Positive—secure, cool, relaxing
	Negative—sad, draining, depressing
Green:	Positive—calming, relaxing, prosperous
	Negative—nauseating, envy
Orange:	Positive—cheerful, friendly, outgoing
	Negative—cheap, gaudy, brassy
Pink:	Positive—young, fun, feminine
	Negative—tacky, pampered, cute, feminine
Red:	Positive—exciting, bold, stimulating
	Negative—aggressive, overpowering, anger
Purple:	Positive—noble, sophisticated, regal, royal
	Negative—pomp, snobbery
Brown:	Positive—homey, earthy, basic
	Negative—sober, dour, uninteresting
White:	Positive—pure, spiritual, clean
	Negative—cold, sterile, blinding

Lighting

Lighting is critical for quality, professional work and to enhance your overall decor. The more lighting the better. A ceiling light and two adjustable arm lamps should be provided for each nail technician table. This combination of light will eliminate error-causing shadows. Other services, particularly skin care, will require other lighting.

Window Treatments

Window treatments should be given careful consideration as to how the choices coordinate with the salon's interior and exterior. Also consider whether or not the products you will be using would be affected by natural or artificial light. This could influence your window treatment options. Think of which colors and textures are used elsewhere in the salon and what type of customer will make up the majority of your clientele. What are their probable likes and dislikes in decor, textures, and colors? For windows, consider levelors with matching wallpaper inserts to give a unique look.

However, the windows should be the last area to finalize. Do some footwork. Look at other salons for ideas. Decide what you like and don't like and consolidate your ideas before you start your own salon.

NEGOTIATIONS

I can just imagine you asking now, "why would I want to read this and why should this be important?" Believe it or not, this is important. Unless you have had specific training in this area, you probably have never thought much about the techniques of negotiation.

Think about it. We negotiate constantly, in all kinds of different situations, such as with our husbands or wives, our children, business acquaintances, people at work, personal acquaintances, officials, salespeople, etc.

Negotiation is defined as to "confer, bargain or discuss with a view to reaching agreement." How we handle ourselves and the effectiveness of our negotiation skills can mean an enormous difference in the outcome of any relationship. You need to develop negotiation skills to become more effective in all your interpersonal relationships and to give yourself an additional competitive business edge. As you deal with landlords, suppliers, salespeople, and customers you will need all the advantages you can get.

The value of effective negotiation is that it prevents lopsided or distorted results; extremes are minimized or avoided. The best "deal" can be achieved, and since all parties contribute to the outcome the results will in all probability be longer lasting.

Negotiation skills are critical for salon owners. Success depends on each party knowing what they want and need and anticipating what the other party wants and needs. Develop a positive problem-solving attitude. There should be no winner and no loser, but rather, a fair settlement both parties can live with. Try to let negotiations continue naturally, at their own pace. You don't need to rush or be in too big a hurry. You should also have alternative suggestions when the issue comes to a stalled point, and use ultimatums only as a last resort. Always leave room for counteroffers until the objectives are achieved.

Negotiation tactics are important, some of which include:

1. Ask for a better deal. Sometimes simply asking will result in a better price, better terms, better quality, or better service.
2. Leave yourself room. Start with greater demands than you expect to achieve. Those who aim higher will do better.
3. Be stingy. Make concessions slowly and grudgingly. Draw out the negotiations by making small concessions.
4. Negotiate with apparent limited authority. Being able to say "if it were up to me" is often an advantage. It gives you time to think, hold tight, and get a better feel for the other person's position. Best of all, it gives the other person a face-saving way to give in.
5. Bite your tongue. The less the other person knows about your motives, limitations, and deadlines the better for you. Get information; don't give it.
6. Competition. If the other person thinks there is competition, then there is competition. Indicate your choices: You can use something new or used, you can buy or do without, etc.
7. Call a time out. If negotiations get bogged down, request time to consult with a partner or lawyer. This will give the other person time to doubt and reconsider and give you time to reaffirm your position or offer a small concession.
8. Beware of quick deals. Give yourself plenty of time to think, to get the whole picture.

9. Surprise. A sudden shift in tone, method, argument, or approach during negotiations can be used to make a point, unsettle the other person, or force a concession.

10. Make a bold move. This is risky but it can be effective in the right situation. For example, if a contract is sent to you with a paragraph you don't like, cross the paragraph out, sign the contract, and return it. Perhaps it will be accepted.

11. No pain, no gain. Make the other person work for every concession you make. The negotiator who gives freely will lose greatly.

12. Use budget tactic. You want it, like it, but can't afford it.

13. Nibble for extras. Small concessions may be important to you but less important to the other person.

14. Be patient. Don't expect instant acceptance. Hold tight, be patient, and your opponent may give in and accept your position or point.

15. Don't corner the other person. Leave room for him or her to save face. There should be no losers, only winners.

Remember, effective negotiating skills properly developed will greatly increase your success as a business owner in today's competitive marketplace.

SUMMARY

There are many steps to be taken and things to consider when you decide to begin a new business. Your salon's location and decor are very important; be sure to investigate thoroughly before signing a lease or making any major purchases. Know as much as possible and have everything put in writing.

Your attorney, accountant, and insurance agent should be selected with the utmost care. Talk to other business owners, check references, and be very selective. These people will be vital to your salon's success, so be certain about their abilities.

A well-thought-out and professional advertising campaign is crucial for a new salon. Research all the possibilities, study your potential clients and demographics, and remember to budget adequately.

EMPLOYEES

C H A P T E R

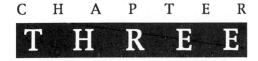

THREE

Your next critical activity will be hiring your employees. There are several positions you may need to fill, including a receptionist, a salon manager, and nail technicians. By conducting a thorough interview, you will make sure the individual has the skills and experience needed to do the job well.

You will need a way to measure and evaluate your employees' performance once they are hired, so that you can form a basis upon which to promote, demote, give raises, or terminate. As an employer, you will also need to know how to deal with employee situations that require discipline, or even termination.

HIRING

Hiring the right people will make or break your business. It is definitely less expensive in every aspect to select the right person than to just hire anyone and suffer the consequences until you are finally forced to take drastic action. By then the damage will have been done in terms of disgruntled customers, poor morale among the staff, and to your financial bottom line.

First, you must prepare a comprehensive job description for each salon position—receptionist, nail technician, other technicians, and even for a manager if you decide to have one. Decide what you want to be performed by each position, in as much detail as possible. Identify what skills, attributes, and duties will be expected for each position. You must then create a questionnaire that addresses and covers the essential qualities and skills you want in an employee. As a minimum, you will want to:

- Check references.
- Acquire a good understanding of the person's work habits, i.e., punctuality, absences, willingness to take on extra work, and personal grooming.
- Acquire an idea of the individual's relationship with coworkers and customers. You must also evaluate the person's interpersonal skills.
- Know the level of technical skills required by the position you are seeking to fill.

Next, you will need a job application form. You can purchase generic printed applications from your local office supply store or you can have a printer prepare your own personally designed application on your letterhead with your logo. I would suggest, if your budget allows, having your own personalized application prepared as it indicates a degree of professionalism to potential employees.

Interviews

If you are not an experienced interviewer I suggest you develop these skills. They are important. How effectively you handle this particular responsibility will have far reaching consequences on your business success.

Before you actually start looking for employees you must carefully think through how you will do your interviews. You need to prepare a "game plan," a process to follow. You want to do as thorough an interview as possible in order to evaluate the prospective employee's ability to meet your previously prepared job description requirements. However, you also do not want to waste your time or that of the person being interviewed. The interview itself is time consuming but invaluable. Be prepared to take as much time as necessary, in a quiet, uninterrupted location, to effectively evaluate the prospective employee.

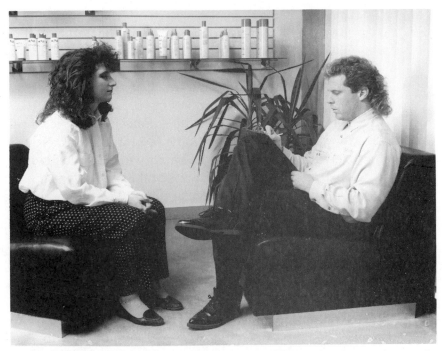

You must do as thorough an interview as possible to determine the candidate's qualifications for the job.

If possible, have someone else whom you trust and respect interview the individual also so you can compare notes and make a better decision. (Hint: always hire smart people.) Some important points to keep in mind are:

1. Be consistent with your interviewing technique and style. Ask each person the same questions, in the same order.
2. Take notes so that you won't forget anything, especially the most important points.
3. Conduct all interviews in private and without interruptions or distractions.
4. Be aware of federal, state, and local laws against job discrimination. In general, you cannot discriminate against anyone because of race, color, sex, age, religion, national origin/ancestry, or physical impairment if the person can perform the job as stated in the job description.

5. Don't ask for information you don't need or can't use. Keep the questions specific to your job description and requirements. Examples of questions you cannot ask: Do you plan on having children? What does your husband do?
6. Concentrate your questions on the applicant's qualifications for the particular job you are seeking to fill.
7. Don't ask questions about the applicant's physical health.
8. You can inquire about training/education as it relates to the specific job, the individual's ability to work the hours required for the position, why the applicant has an interest in working for you, specific skills, and the applicant's willingness to demonstrate technical ability.

As part of your standard hiring procedures I would recommend you hire on a trial basis, i.e., for two to three months. This gives you an "out" in case the individual just doesn't measure up to your original evaluation. No matter how good your interviewing skills and techniques, you will not be able to tell everything you need to know about an individual from your interview. Once you decide to offer an individual a position with your salon, be sure to explain, in detail, your expectations of employees and your salon policies and procedures.

There are several sources for identifying potential applicants, the most obvious being cosmetology schools, local schools with job placement services, current customers, and newspaper want ads. If you do advertise for applicants, keep the ad short and simple, with a minimum of information to outline the basics of the position. Let the ad do some of the "weeding out" process of unqualified applicants.

For the exceptional applicant, you may have to sell yourself and your salon to get the individual onto your staff. Be prepared to discuss what you and your salon have to offer this individual, such as:

- Competitive salary/income.
- An established clientele.
- Good salon location, parking, safe neighborhood.
- Pleasant salon atmosphere and friendly coworkers.
- Continuing education.
- Salon staff library with the latest books, trade newspapers, and magazines.
- Sales incentive program.

- Aggressive advertising programs for new customer development.
- Insurance, vacations, etc.
- Anything else you can think of that would sell your salon.

Once you have hired an individual, you must personally train the individual in the new position, regardless of how much experience or training the person has. This individual will represent you and your salon to your clientele so you do not want to delegate this responsibility to anyone else. This is your best opportunity to instill in everyone you hire the way in which you want your salon to be operated and the standards to be maintained.

Your salon reputation will be built by your staff. Keep them well supervised, yet happy. If you are fair and continually boost their morale, you will be rewarded by high profits and a great, successful salon.

Receptionist

I would strongly recommend you consider having a receptionist for your salon. The benefits derived by having a good individual in this position can be substantial. The receptionist can free you and the technicians of many responsibilities, which means everyone can be more productive for the salon. A good receptionist makes customers feel good and important, from the time they first telephone your salon to when they leave the salon with another appointment booked. The receptionist helps the entire salon run more smoothly.

Hiring the right individual is very important. To be a good receptionist an individual should genuinely like people and be able to make a good first impression. The person should exhibit an eagerness to learn, be consistently pleasant, and have an even disposition and professional demeanor. Your receptionist must be able to handle angry or unhappy customers without getting emotional; be honest, dependable, and responsible; and exhibit a genuine enjoyment for the job. Look for someone who is a good speaker with excellent telephone etiquette. And be sure your receptionist is very well groomed (hair, nails, makeup, and fragrance).

The receptionist's duties and responsibilities should include:

- Knowledge of the salon products and services in order to be able to answer questions related to the salon services and staff.

- Handle sales receipts, cash, checks, cash register.
- Maintain technicians' appointment books, which would include being familiar with the technicians' schedules and areas of expertise and how long each takes to do a particular service.
- Set up and maintain the retail area.
- Handle some bookkeeping, banking, inventory, and ordering of supplies.
- Ability to remain calm in a crisis.
- Good with customer relations—making sure reading material is available, providing refreshments, etc.
- Handle mailings to customers, reminder notices to old clients, and thank-you notes to new customers.
- Maintain a waiting list for cancellation fill-ins.
- Remind customers of the salon cancellation policy.

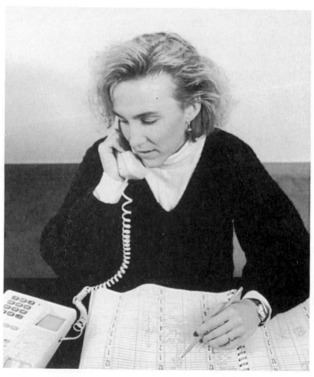

A receptionist helps the entire salon run more smoothly.

Once you have selected your receptionist, be sure to personally and thoroughly train the individual in exactly how you expect her to perform her duties. This should not be delegated to anyone else. Remember, the receptionist gives the first and last impression of your salon to your customers.

Salon Manager

At some time or another, you will think about wanting or needing a salon manager to help you out. When that time comes, what should you consider? Remember, your salon has taken on your individual personality and you must be very careful who you consider for this position.

First, as with all positions, you must prepare a job description. What would you want a manager to do? What are your personal management strengths and weaknesses? You will need someone to complement your style, not duplicate your strong and weak traits. You will want someone who will fill a need as you define that need, not just someone to fill a space on an organization chart.

You must decide what hours this person will work; what technical and other special skills you require; and what jobs this person will perform, such as conducting meetings, educating the staff, and customer relations. When selecting a manager, remember that it is extremely difficult to change someone's basic personality and biases. It is easier to search for the individual who best fits your requirements than to put just anyone in the position and hope to change or train her to fulfill your expectations. In addition, always choose an optimist, a person with a healthy and positive outlook, who is a natural winner.

When interviewing, ask each applicant the same set of questions, take notes, and don't jump around with your questions. Be consistent. Then when you have finished with all the applicants, you can make a good solid informed judgment. You want a manager who can be a natural leader, who can inspire others, who will listen and be able to manage in a positive, constructive manner. Most of all you want a manager who is honest. You might consider the following questions to generate the responses you need for your evaluation:

- What kind of individual would you consider the best boss?
- What kind of work situation/environment would you consider the ideal?

- How would you manage a salon?
- What did you like best about your last two jobs? What did you like the least?
- What gets you excited? What motivates you?
- What kind of people do you like the best? The least? Why?
- How would you handle customers, staff, problem situations, taking responsibility, conflict, stressful situations?

The biggest mistake you can make is to try and make a manager out of someone who really isn't a manager. Also, be very careful about considering good friends for this position. Remember, business is business and friends are friends. Be very careful and selective about the individual you place in this position.

Technicians

Once you have decided on which services you want to provide and how large a salon you want, you will need to consider hiring your technicians. For discussion purposes, let's assume you are starting out as a one-person salon. You will need to hire your first technician when your bookings reach 75 percent of your available time. Then with your customer base continually increasing, your next staff increase should be when the bookings again reach 75 percent of your combined available time.

There are two types of employees you can hire—skilled and unskilled. Personally, I always enjoyed training new people without any prior experience. In my state this was necessary most of the time because the nail trade is unlicensed and the availability of good, experienced technicians is always a problem. Even if I hire "skilled" technicians I always retrain them to meet my standards, which are very high. I find it easier to train someone completely new instead of retraining someone else by having to change their old work habits and skills. Besides, by doing the training and teaching the way I want the service provided to the customer I guarantee uniformity among the staff and the adherence of high-quality standards.

The advantage to hiring skilled technicians is that you may not have to do too much retraining. The individual can start work and earn income more quickly. Also, in some instances experienced technicians may have their own customers who will follow them to your salon.

In addition to technical skills, your technicians should have pleasing appearances and personalities and enjoy working with people. They should be cooperative and willing to commit to the overall objectives of the salon and be willing to learn new skills and techniques as required.

PERFORMANCE REVIEWS AND SALARY ADJUSTMENTS

Now you need a systematic approach to measuring and evaluating your employees' performance. This performance evaluation will be the basis for your decisions regarding any possible salary compensation adjustments, promotions, demotions, or terminations. A structured performance evaluation process will be the basis for offering guidance, instruction, encouragement, and motivation to the employee.

Objectives/Goals

First, for each separate position within the salon you must have established a formal job description and a list of duties.

Next, for each employee you must establish objectives or goals to be achieved. These are to be statements of the specific results expected during the next appraisal period for each of the major duties. Most employees will have at least four objectives and should have no more than eight. If there are more than eight, it's likely you have defined the objectives/goals too narrowly. An objective should:

1. Clearly state the specific results expected, such as reaching a certain income level, maintaining a level of quality of work, or adhering to salon policies and procedures.
2. Be realistic and obtainable.
3. Represent acceptable performance.
4. Be measurable.

Objectives need to specify what is to be done, when or within what time frames, and how or under what conditions. Objectives should indicate the broad parameters within which the results need to be accomplished.

Standards of Performance

Next, you will need to define standards of performance that must be achieved to meet each of your performance levels. Standards may be qualitative, quantitative, or a combination of the two.

Qualitative standards reflect the quality of the result, which often can't be precisely measured and generally will reflect your judgment. Quantitative standards are measured in numbers—number of customer complaints, number of sets completed in a given time frame, number of new customers. For performance standards I would suggest five levels:

1. Significantly exceeds acceptable performance
2. Exceeds acceptable performance
3. Meets acceptable performance
4. Falls short of acceptable performance
5. Falls significantly short of acceptable performance

All standards must be attainable. Even the standard for performance level one must be realistic, though it must necessarily represent an ambitious goal. Also, the standard for performance level five should be specified. It isn't sufficient to just say "unacceptable performance." The standard should specify what results are unacceptable.

To develop standards, start with a thorough definition of acceptable performance for level three. Then, working from this definition, specify standards at levels one, five, two, and four.

Measurements

The next step is to identify measurements that you will use to evaluate the employee's performance. For instance, if one of your standards is five new customers a week, agree on how these new customers are to be identified so that there will not be any misunderstanding when the evaluation process begins.

Prior to the evaluation period, or at the beginning of the evaluation period, you and the employee must agree on the objectives/goals, the standards, and the measurements so that there will not be any misunderstandings at the end of the evaluation period when the performance of the employee is evaluated.

By having job descriptions and a structured, standardized performance evaluation process administered fairly and uniformly you protect yourself from unlawful employee termination. Let your attorney review your program for advice from a legal perspective. Besides, it's simply more businesslike to have a formal program than to just "fly by the seat of your pants."

Schedules

It is important that you administer appraisals and evaluations on a scheduled routine basis, usually every six months for each employee. Consider annual review with an interim review every three months. Everyone wants to be recognized for doing a good job and for improving one's overall skill level. As corny as it sounds, a happy employee is much more likely to be a productive employee. You can also prevent a disgruntled employee from having a negative effect on the morale of the rest of the staff.

Be sure to schedule the performance evaluation session with sufficient notice to the employee. Don't just one day surprise the employee by announcing that it's time for the performance review. Give the employee at least one week's notice of the day and time the review will be held. Ask the employee to do his/her own performance evaluation so you can discuss any differences of opinion and resolve any misunderstandings.

Review Session

Be sure to allow plenty of uninterrupted time for the review session. Don't rush through the session but be sincerely interested in each employee and the performance review process. Demonstrate that you care for high-quality standards and due recognition. This is a good time for the practice of your listening skills.

Be sure to conduct the performance review session in private. You don't want interruptions and you certainly wouldn't want to violate the confidentiality of the employee's performance evaluation.

Remember, you are the boss and you must take the lead to set the tone for the meeting. Be natural and put the employee at ease so that the session can be as relaxed as possible. Begin by explaining and reviewing the purpose of the session. Explain again your performance review evaluation program, why it was established, and how it is administered.

You need to be formal, fair, and realistic as you go through the evaluation; be specific and to say what you mean. This is not the time for small talk or daily chatter. Be objective and keep the process on a positive and constructive level. Always be encouraging.

Above all, be fair and consistent with your performance evaluations. You do not want to give one employee the same evaluation or grade for doing more or less than you gave another employee for the same job performance. But if an employee has performed well and accomplished the goals by all means be fair and give recognition for the accomplishment.

At the conclusion of the review you and the employee must agree on the evaluation (or at least agree on what was discussed) and you both should add any comments and sign the review form. You should also discuss and agree upon the objectives and goals for the new upcoming review period. Reach an agreement with the employee as to what will be expected, the standards for the objectives, and how the standards will be measured. Agree when the next interim review will be conducted.

Salary Adjustments and Promotions

As mentioned earlier, performance reviews should be completed at least every six months. However, any adjustment to salary (raises) and/or promotions should be done only on an annual basis.

An individual doesn't automatically get an increase in pay for doing a satisfactory job. That's what the individual is paid for in the first place. However, an exceptionally good job and/or an increase in skill levels should be recognized and rewarded. A salary adjustment should indicate excellent work, progress or accomplishment of specific goals and objectives, or increased responsibilities.

COMPENSATION ALTERNATIVES   There are compensation alternatives, other than money, for recognition following a performance review. Different forms of recognition are extremely effective, for example certificates, awards, or press releases. Increased benefits are also effective. Or, the employee could be given the opportunity to attend an employer-paid class, seminar, or trade exhibit. For some individuals a more liberal and flexible work schedule would be an excellent reward alternative. An effective employee performance review program is critical for a successful business. You must take the responsibility to make sure it happens.

Motivation is the psychological condition of wanting to do something. Performance is doing something according to specific expectations and/or standards. Most employees want to do a good job and usually those who don't measure up do not because they don't understand clearly what is expected of them. It is usually a communication issue. Another reason is the lack of regular and specific feedback from their manager/boss.

Important Reminders

- Establish job descriptions, standards and measurements for each position in the salon.
- Schedule routine appraisals/evaluations for each employee.
- Prepare carefully for each performance review meeting. Review the last performance evaluation. Make a list of the items you want to discuss and be sure to note all positive aspects of the performance, not just negative issues.
- Review the purpose for the meeting with the employee, what you want to accomplish, your performance review program, and how it works.
- Listen carefully and ask clarifying questions. Be patient.
- Avoid personal criticism. Stick to the issue—the review of the individual's performance during the appraisal period.
- During the meeting, summarize from time to time to make sure you understand what you're hearing, what conclusions were reached, and to make sure that there are not any misunderstandings.
- Be courteous, sincere, businesslike, and show interest.
- Conclude with a summary and a plan mutually agreed upon to address any issues that were identified as needing attention, i.e., better interpersonal skills, better work quality, or faster work.

REMUNERATION

When it comes to remuneration for technicians, you have several choices:

1. Paying a straight hourly salary
2. Paying a salary on a guaranteed amount plus commission

3. Paying straight commission
4. Renting stations or space to technicians
5. A combination of rental and commission

Hourly Salary

The straight hourly salary is the simplest method to administer and must conform to the federal minimum wage level. The main drawback to a straight salary is the lack of incentive for the technician to do as much work as possible. But there are some advantages for the salon owner, such as having someone available during set hours for walk-ins or emergencies. Under this remuneration arrangement the salon owner usually provides all the equipment, supplies, and advertising. The technician usually provides work equipment, such as brushes.

Salary Plus Commission

The second method, paying a minimum salary plus a commission, is especially good for use with the less experienced technician while she is building up clientele. The technician must first double the base amount (salary) then everything over that doubled amount is commissioned at an agreed upon percentage. For example, if the employee worked forty hours and the hourly rate was $5, the salary would be $200. Double this to get the $400 base. If the employee produced $600 in service income to the salon, $200 ($600 minus $400) times the agreed upon commission rate would be earned.

Commission

Once the technician has achieved a certain customer base and level of income, it is in the salon owner's (and employee's) best interest to go to a straight commission schedule. This can be progressive, for example 40 percent for all work up to $500 of service income; 45 percent if the volume ranges between $500 and $600; 50 percent for everything above $600. The percentage depends on how much you can afford to pay, if you provide any supplies, and what the local going commission rate is. Many variations and combinations can be utilized.

Renting Stations

Renting stations to technicians is in my opinion not a desirable option. Under this agreement, the technician would be considered an independent contractor, not an employee. **CAUTION**: Be sure to discuss this with your attorney.

Normally, a technician renting space from a salon supplies his or her own furniture, telephone, advertising, supplies, towels, insurance, laundering—just about everything. However, this is all subject to negotiation. The technician would also, normally, set his or her own working hours.

A major drawback of this arrangement (from your perspective) could be an individual's reluctance to participate in staff meetings. The technician also may not have a vested interest in teamwork or anything else that you want your salon to represent. The individual could become extremely independent and you wouldn't have any control whatsoever, so long as he or she lived up to the rental agreement. Morale could become a major problem as you would simply not be in control. I would strongly advise against this arrangement for a salon owner interested in a first class salon with high professional standards.

But if you do find a situation where it is advantageous to rent space, make sure your lease allows you to sublet, because this is in fact what you are doing. (If you are a technician wanting to rent/lease space in a salon, there are other considerations you have to be aware of, such as having to do your own bookkeeping, inventory, and taxes. It is a lot to consider and could become a major headache.)

About the only time I would recommend that you consider renting out space is when you have a technician with a specialty that you don't know anything about but would like to add to your list of services. An example would be a full-service nail salon with an opportunity to add a hair stylist, or something similar. You will have to weigh the advantages against the disadvantages in such a situation.

A strong word of caution: Anytime you decide to rent out station space to a technician, it is critical that all terms of the agreement be agreed upon by all parties and that everything be put in writing by the salon owner, building management, and the technician renting the space. Whoever handles the receipts and payroll must also be aware of the arrangement. Needless to say, work with your attorney so that the contract completely represents the agreement.

Rental/Commission

The fifth method is a combination of both rental and commission. Again, the exact specifics of the arrangement are fully negotiable and can be as varied as the situation warrants.

Under the right circumstance, each of these options offer advantages to the salon owner. And it is quite possible that several types of compensation plans will be in effect at the same time. In other words, you may have one technician on a straight guaranteed salary, and others may be on straight commission.

Holiday Pay/Bonuses

Holiday pay, either higher commission or bonuses, is very effective in providing incentives for technicians. For example, if you have a commission schedule that pays 45 percent for a $500 week and 50 percent for a $600 week, increase each range by $2\frac{1}{2}$ to 5 percent to encourage the staff to work longer hours. The same goes for retail sales. Set an acceptable or realistic volume of sales for the salon and pay a 10 percent bonus to the employees for everything above this amount. (Once established, the volume can become your twelve-month average and be used in future bonus programs.) Prepare a sales chart so everyone can monitor the progress of the sales activity increases to keep interest high. Post this in a nonpublic area, such as in the employee break area or lounge.

Tipping

Tipping has been around for a long time. Some business owners consider it a problem and discourage it. Others encourage tipping and even consider it a part of the employee compensation package. Many technicians increase their income significantly from tips and guard their better tipping customers most carefully. This is one subject that most technicians do not talk about among themselves (except for poor tipping customers). You as a salon owner should encourage this at all times; employees should not discuss the tipping habits of customers. The subject of tipping and certainly the amount of tips is simply not a topic of conversation in the salon. You do need to establish a salon policy on whether or not you will allow tipping. I find it encourages the staff to perform better service for the customers.

The Internal Revenue Service (IRS), however, takes quite another view of tipping. They expect all tips to be reported as income and taxes paid accordingly. This is the individual employee's responsibility but you as an owner should remind your staff of their obligation. You should also remind your staff to keep good records of their tips and to complete the appropriate IRS reporting forms. Again, check with your accountant or attorney for full compliance procedures.

As an employer, you must withhold Social Security tax and any income tax due on tips reported to you by your employees. The amount withheld is to be subtracted from the employees' wages unless an exception is claimed.

EMPLOYMENT CONTRACTS

I have used employment contracts with some of my technicians. In the beauty business, customer loyalty is oftentimes more with the technician than with a particular salon or salon owner. As much as you work to prevent this it will still exist. If you have hired and trained the best people then you will want to do everything possible to retain and protect your investment.

An employment contract provides a clear understanding in writing, that can be referred to at anytime, of what was originally agreed upon. Misunderstandings, disputes, hard feelings, morale issues are reduced by such a contract. Anything and everything (that's legal) between the contracting parties can and should be in an employment agreement, including:

- Working hours
- Overtime policy
- Termination
- Training
- Duties/responsibilities
- Who provides what, i.e., supplies
- Method of compensation
- Benefits
- Promotions
- Vacations
- Adherence to salon policies and procedures.

Let's face facts though; you cannot force anyone to work for you and do a good job if they do not want to. Situations change and sometimes people do too. You as an employer would not want to continue with an employee against your will, so I would recommend a clause that allows either yourself or the employee to terminate the contract at any time for any reason. However, you can build into the contract a provision that, for considerations provided, if the employee terminates the contract there would be a no-compete agreement for a certain reasonable period of time (one year) within a certain geographic area (ten-mile radius of your salon). You might also want to consider a clause prohibiting the ex-employee from soliciting your customers. Also, consider arbitration clauses for settling disputes. Again, see your attorney for guidance and advice.

BURNOUT

Many people are subject to job burnout at one time or another. Any job that exhausts you emotionally and physically can eventually burn you out. You need to guard against this personally and be sensitive to it in your employees. People who are self-driven, goal-oriented, perfectionist over-achievers with high expectations for themselves and others are prime candidates for burnout. Burnout can surface as anger, depression, irritability, poor work quality, impatience, indifference, tardiness, physical exhaustion, or any number of emotional reactions.

If you suspect burnout is a real issue you must take steps to address the situation quickly before serious results occur. There are many things you can do. First, whether with yourself or an employee you must try to identify the real cause. Be honest with your evaluation so you can determine what can be done to correct the problem. Assuming it isn't medically or physically based, you should be able to come up with any number of ideas to put new vigor into your lifestyle—anything from a vacation to a new leisure activity such as watching sunsets.

If the burnout seems to be affecting the salon staff as a whole you might consider something to put new excitement into your salon routine. Be creative:

- Have a salon "theme" day to break the routine.
- Develop holiday or promotional specials.
- Have an employee incentive campaign.
- Have a "wine and bagels" night.
- Add new flowers to the salon.
- Start an employee recognition program.
- Look for things to do differently, or by different employees.

If you suspect burnout, step back and review your situation. Think of ways to change your activities and involvements. Do something different. On a personal level be sure to exercise, rest, eat properly, and stay healthy.

DISCIPLINE

As a business owner, there will be times when you have to discipline an employee because of any number of reasons, such as absenteeism, incompetence, poor morale, or failure to comply with the salon rules and regulations. Your job is to address the situation quickly before it gets out of hand and becomes a larger problem requiring drastic action.

When you do find yourself in a situation requiring discipline, you must prepare to move quickly. Have a meeting with the employee in private and ask questions in order to allow the employee to give her side of the situation. Be calm and in control. Don't lose your temper and don't deliberately provoke the other person. You both should agree as to what the problem is and what the employee will do to correct the situation. Explain exactly what you expect, and if appropriate, time frames in which it should be done. Reach an agreement and an understanding.

If this is the first incident, you might want to put a short informal summary of the discussion in the employee's personnel file. If this is a second occurrence of the same problem the discussion should be formalized in detail, in writing, with expectations clearly spelled out, signed, and dated. Remember, this is your business and you must protect it.

TERMINATION

Although this is not a pleasant subject, it is necessary because at some point you will be forced to terminate an employee. Your business interests must come first to you, even if it means terminating a friend. A good manager will create a work environment that encourages all employees to be as responsible as they can be, but the basic responsibility of an owner is to ensure that the job gets done and that responsibilities are fulfilled.

Assuming that you have provided each employee with a job description for her particular position and a handbook or guideline of your salon's rules and regulations, and that you have conducted regular performance reviews in a positive and constructive manner, the difficultly of terminating someone has been largely minimized.

When you start to have problems with an employee, meet with her to discuss it honestly and openly. Outline the problem as you understand it and agree on a solution. If the problem continues, have another meeting but put everything in writing, with both of you signing the review and put the review in the personnel file.

If you have done everything you should have done as a good manager/owner—established job descriptions; prepared a salon procedures manual; held regular staff meetings; conducted periodic one-on-one employee performance reviews; provided the equipment, supplies, and training for the job—then you do not and should not feel guilty if an employee doesn't do her part and you must terminate her.

Carefully rehearse what you are going to say to the employee prior to the meeting and how you will say it. Practice your comments. Prepare for the anticipated employee reaction and for your response. Anticipate emotional reactions (if it's not a favorable review) so as not to be swayed from your decision. Be as short and simple as possible, make your points, and stick with your decision. Have your discussion in private and without interruptions. If possible, have a witness or someone else not directly involved sit in during a particularly sensitive or difficult meeting.

Some managers believe in telling an employee they are termininated and having the employee leave the salon as quietly and as quickly as possible. Others believe in giving the employee time to finish up whatever she is doing and to say goodbye. I personally believe in the "quiet and quick" policy in order to avoid disruption of the salon business.

Finally, don't argue, don't insult, don't admit that you are sorry, and don't give the individual any false hope that you may change your mind. Most important, don't feel guilty. If you've done everything to the best of your ability, you certainly should not have to feel any guilt. As unpleasant as it is to terminate someone, sometimes it just has to be done. It is part of business.

SUMMARY

Your employees must reflect the image and professionalism of your salon. Select them very carefully, keep them well supervised, and reward or reprimand them as necessary. Comprehensive job descriptions and thorough interviewing procedures will help you to choose the right people. Proper training will assure that they perform up to your standards.

You will need to determine what form of remuneration you will use for each of your employees and implement a procedure for periodic performance reviews and salary adjustments. Be prepared to discipline employees when the need arises, and always be on the lookout for signs of job burnout, in yourself or your employees.

Proper training and communication is vital to your employees' job performance. Still, there may come a time when you will have to terminate someone. Be prepared for this and do it quickly and professionally.

SALON OPERATIONS

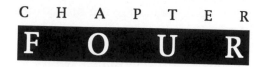
Many day-to-day operations are necessary to maintain a smooth regularity in your salon. Setting guidelines as to salon attire and behavior are important steps to keep your professional image. By holding regular, planned staff meetings you will keep on top of employee concerns and heighten communication. Making sure your employees have access to training will ensure that they (and you) will stay abreast of changes in techniques and products.

Ordering supplies, deciding on a shipper for your orders, dealing with returned checks from customers, and resolving customer complaints are many other things that need to be dealt with during the day's operations. Are you familiar with how to handle these situations?

MANAGEMENT

Times and attitudes as regards employer/employee relationships have changed dramatically during the last few decades. The carrot-and-the-stick mentality is history. No longer is it appropriate to model the energy-consuming task of disciplining unwanted behavior and reinforcing wanted behavior. You should strive to create a dynamic environment where an individual's natural, innate abilities flourish. Salon owners today must be leaders instead of old-fashioned bosses. Fear and reward is no longer effective.

Modern employees expect far more from a job than just a pay check. They want a sense of belonging, a feeling of self-respect, a chance for advancement, a pride in accomplishment, and the opportunity for social status and recognition.

Your Responsibilities

You as an owner or manager must recognize these changes and be prepared to address them. Everything reasonable must be done to maintain a high level of morale and to keep staff turnover at a minimum.

You as an owner must keep motivated employees performing up to your expectations and standards. You must ensure satisfactory performance and not allow your actions to be an impediment. You must give the employee regular and constructive performance feedback; keep lines of communication open; make timely decisions; and be accessible, encouraging, and supportive.

In addition, you as an owner must practice what you preach, i.e., to always set an example. This may be harder to do than you think, but it can be done. Try to always think through your actions before you respond so you won't have to be spending time doing "damage control" after the fact. This is particularly important with all personnel issues.

PERSONAL RESPONSIBILITIES   Your personal responsibilities go beyond dressing for success and always wearing envious nails. You must always leave your personal problems outside the salon door and focus your undivided attention on your clients and staff. You must be confident of your own technical skills and those of your staff; keep a friendly and open rapport with your staff; and have positive, meaningful, and constructive staff meetings.

Personally, you must manage your limited time by prioritizing on a daily basis the items that must be accomplished. Do this the first thing each day. What you don't accomplish today, add to tomorrow's list. Evaluate your own habits and eliminate unproductive routines or activities. Constantly be sensitive to improving your time efficiency. Set deadlines for yourself and keep a record of your progress.

TRAINING

Always make training time available for your staff and for yourself in order to stay abreast of changes in techniques and products. You do not want to shortchange your salon's success by falling behind from an information perspective—doctors, attorneys, and dentists don't; as a professional you can't either.

One good technique is to bring in outside trainers or guest speakers several times a year. Schedule specialists in the training areas needed most by your staff. This means you will have to continually survey and be aware of their needs, such as with nail sculpturing, nail tips, wraps, pedicuring, or waxing. And don't overlook other areas that may need strengthening, such as interpersonal skills, customer relations, or telephone skills. Schedule selected individuals to attend trade shows to learn what is new and to teach the rest of the salon personnel. I would recommend that you close the salon for this type of training but have someone available to answer the telephone so as to prevent interruptions and distractions.

STAFF MEETINGS

Regular, planned staff meetings are a must if you want your salon to succeed and to keep morale high among the staff. To run a tight, efficient operation you must communicate with your staff constantly and effectively to let them know what you expect and how you expect objectives to be achieved.

I found the best way to accomplish my objectives was to create a trusting environment where creative thoughts and ideas were encouraged and where the staff was encouraged to participate without fear of embarrassment.

Effective Meetings

To achieve effective meetings you must know how to conduct them in the most efficient manner. You will want to avoid a lecture-type format where you are in front doing all the talking. Instead, you will want to be more of a facilitator, to make the whole process easier and more productive. In order to be a successful facilitator, you must:

1. Identify how the meeting fits into the overall plan dealing with the issue at hand. For example, is this a meeting to update, educate, identify, or solve a problem?
2. Create a climate that stimulates participation by group members. Start out by going around the room and asking for input from everyone on some aspect of the issue.
3. Understand the problem, task or, issue. If you are not sure, your employees certainly won't be.
4. Plan the process for the meeting as carefully as the content to be discussed.
5. Define the role of the participants—to listen, to give ideas, or to formulate a plan.
6. Be specific about what decisions need to be made and summarize the progress of the meeting at regular intervals.
7. Clearly differentiate between process (here's how we will discuss the topics) and content (now let's begin discussing the topic).
8. Be skilled in questioning techniques that facilitate gathering information on the issues.

An effective meeting starts with the facilitator explaining the purposes and goals of the meeting. In addition to verbally outlining the purposes and goals, the facilitator should write them on a flip chart that is visible to the group throughout the meeting.

AGENDA   Always have an agenda for the meeting. Be sure to ask the group for their input on the agenda items either before the meeting or at the very start of the meeting. Gain the groups agreement as to the agenda items. Having an agenda ensures that there will be no surprises during the meeting. Depending on the circumstances and type of meeting, you might want to distribute the agenda to the group prior to the meeting so that everyone can be familiar with what will be discussed. When reviewing the agenda at the beginning of the meeting, the facilitator gains agreement from the group on the amount of time to be spent on each topic and even on the order of the agenda topics. Try to structure the agenda so that the fun, lighthearted topics are covered first and you progress to the more difficult topics. If possible, try to end the meeting on a light note.

Always start the meeting on a positive note. One good idea is to start with everyone sharing with the group at least one good positive statement or positive example since the last meeting. For example, someone acquired three new customers or someone doubled their retail sale average.

HOLIDAY SEASONS Staff meetings are particularly important prior to the busy and hectic holiday seasons, particularly Christmas, Easter, and Valentine's Day. Your staff must know what you expect of them. They must know you appreciate and understand the strain of working longer hours. They need to know that they must do their own shopping early and organize their own personal schedules to accommodate the extra working hours. At this time you may have to delegate additional responsibilities, such as salon decorations or advertising. Be sure to stress the maintenance of superior customer service and high-quality work. You certainly want to avoid any deterioration of these important items.

YOUR ROLE When conducting a meeting, you are not there to dominate but to encourage individual interactions and to facilitate group discussions. You want to help with reaching decisions, not make them. Avoid leading the meeting, except when opening and closing. As a facilitator, you want to ask questions, to achieve consensus, to give recognition, to keep the meeting agenda on track, and to provide pertinent salon information when necessary. Avoid controlling or overly managing the meeting. As the facilitator you will want to listen more than you talk. Strive for an air of equality, respect, and dignity.

Always express your expectation for the meeting and outline to the group their responsibility toward accomplishing the goal or purpose of the meeting. You will achieve more from your staff if they are involved and play an active and real role in developing solutions instead of simply being on the receiving end of management directives. Try it; you will find that in the long run participative and open meetings really work better.

To make your meetings even more effective try using visual aids, such as flip charts, graphs, or wall posters. Also consider using outside guest speakers, such as distributors, or industry professionals. Demonstrations are also quite effective when introducing new products or techniques.

DIFFICULT EMPLOYEES   From time to time, you may have a difficult employee who tries to dominate the meeting or avoid contributing to the meeting. Don't let these employees take over. I have found that asking other people questions, avoiding eye contact with the difficult individual, and shifting subject matter helps to minimize the problem. Usually the situation can be improved by a one-on-one session with the individual after the meeting to explain the problem, as I see it, and to solicit a more cooperative attitude.

For the employee who won't participate or contribute, again have a one-on-one session and find out what the problem is, if any. Explain that everyone must contribute and that everyone can have constructive input. During the group meeting, ask these noncontributors questions to draw them into the conversation. Once they begin to be a part of the group it's usually smooth sailing from then one.

SALON ATTIRE

In addition to your salon location and decor, your professional image should be enhanced by how you and your staff dress. You do not want a contradiction between you, your salon decor, and the image you project. One unplanned element (attire) could compromise your entire effort.

Dress Code

There are acceptable standards for dressing and acting as a professional in today's competitive, demanding business environment. You, as the owner, must establish a firm but fair dress code. At the same time, however, you must allow for flexibility, to relax the dress code at specified times, such as if you have a theme-related day to tie-in with promotions or for special days such as holidays.

Remember, having nails done is not a necessity, but a luxury. Customers will expect and want technicians who take care of themselves, not someone who looks unkempt. They want a professional in every sense of the word.

An employee must look good to be successful. You, as the owner, need to remind employees that tips can be, and probably will be, a significant part of their earnings. These earnings will be enhanced by superior service, a pleasant rapport between the customer and the technician, and a professional image.

You must establish, as part of your salon procedures manual, a clearly written statement of what you expect from your staff in the way of clothes, style of dressing, and personal demeanor. You have four options:

1. No salon dress policy— everyone dresses as they choose
2. The utilization of lab coats or smocks over street clothes
3. Uniforms
4. A structured dress code for everyone

Believe me, you do not want the first option. You would be amazed at what some people would wear and try to get away with. Lab coats or smocks are a better idea and provide a professional image. The individual's clothing is protected and personal clothing choice is still maintained.

Don't dismiss uniforms lightly. Their utilization should be seriously considered. Today's manufacturers offer a vast improvement over yesterday's styles, colors, and fabrics. Today's choices are fashion conscious with an awareness for styles, fit, color, and fabric. Uniforms also come in dresses; two-pieces; and pants, top, and jacket combinations. Uniforms can be considered as a "perk" for the employee, which would of course become part of your overhead operating expenses. The most important aspect of uniforms is their consistency.

Whatever you do, you must have a dress code. Even if you choose to go with uniforms you must have guidelines. Put in writing exactly what you will and will not allow and stick to it. You should not allow:

Jeans	Bare legs with
Shorts	dresses or skirts
Sandals	Sockless feet
Tennis shoes	Miniskirts
Tank tops	Tight pants
Oversized or	Sweatsuits or
clunky jewelry	exercise attire

You need to consider the following when establishing your dress code:

- If in doubt, don't wear it.
- Sleeves should not be too long (they can get ruined or soiled).

- Necklines should not gape in front.
- High-necked blouses should not choke when you are bending over.
- Shoulder movements should not be restricted.
- Skirts should not hike up too much when you sit down.
- Skirts/slacks should be loose enough for long periods of sitting.
- Hosiery is required by many state regulators and should be worn for hygienic and esthetic purposes.
- Hair and makeup should be appropriate for a professional image.

You should also set out guidelines to address chewing gum, excessive perfumes, and other personal scents. If you rent stations to technicians, the rental contract should include guidelines to comply with your salon dress code. If you don't put it in writing you will not have any recourse, except moral persuasion, and your salon image could be severely compromised.

TRADE SHOWS

Trade shows have become very large and popular. Today they are being held throughout the year around the country. I have found trade shows to be fun, interesting, and educational. You can also get good buys on new products. By attending trade shows you are giving yourself the opportunity to stay abreast of the latest in techniques and new products.

Attending trade shows is also an excellent "perk" for your outstanding employees and helps to keep staff interest and morale high. You should keep this in mind during your performance reviews and when you are preparing your annual budget.

Plan your trip so that your time is well spent. Know what you want to accomplish before you leave for the show. Do you want to view products new to the market, talk to suppliers of products you use, question suppliers of products you may be interested in using, or visit with other salon owners? How much you accomplish at a trade show depends upon how well you plan your time and activities. Set your goals and objectives on paper. For the trip itself:

- Call the show manager in advance for a list of exhibitors, hotels that offer discounts, show times, etc.

- Book your travel and air fare in advance to save money.
- Travel with a companion for safety and to save on cab and hotel expenses.
- Buy presale show tickets to save money.
- Take an envelope for all receipts and note on each one what it was for (you will need this at income tax time).
- Wear comfortable shoes and dress conservatively.
- Don't wear expensive jewelry.
- Carry a briefcase instead of a purse.
- Be aware of criminals and thieves at all such industry shows. Be careful and don't draw attention to yourself.
- Bring a large supply of business cards.
- Bring a pad of paper and pen for notes.

Once you get to the show, go to the information desk to get a copy of the show program. Identify the exhibitors you want to see, the restaurants, and rest rooms. Locate and circle each one on a map if one is provided. Get your bearings. Plan your activities for the best and most economical way to see everything you want to see. Work out your own schedule and itinerary.

SHIPPING

Another expense item to consider in order to have a more favorable bottom line is your shipping costs. We all understand how it works—we place an order, the supplier then contracts with a shipper to deliver the order, and we pay for it. But problems can occur if the order is incomplete, wrong, or if there has been any damage. What can you do?

First, you can negotiate with the supplier to use the shipper of your choice. Watch costs closely and shop around to determine how you can secure the lowest rates.

When accepting your order always try to inspect the items before you sign for them. If you can't do this because you or the delivery person doesn't have time, then write next to your signature that you are accepting the shipment uninspected. If it's because the delivery person can't or won't wait, note that. If you see any sign of damage or abuse, such as a damaged container, rattling contents, or anything abnormal, note it when you sign your name and have the delivery person make a note as well. If the delivery person refuses to let you inspect the contents or won't note any abnormalities, don't accept the shipment. You could have damaged goods with a poor chance for recovery. Also, get the name of the delivery company and the delivery person and notify the shipper of any problems or concerns.

For COD (cash on delivery) orders, you should definitely insist on inspecting the merchandise before you pay for it. If you do not and there is a problem with the shipment, you could have more difficulty in getting any satisfaction. Always check the amount of freight charged on your invoice with the amount on the bill of lading for accuracy. Mistakes can happen, and not necessarily in your favor.

BOUNCED CHECKS

Let's face it, for a business this is a fact of life. From time to time you will get a customer's check back from your bank. What do you do?

First, it is vital that you have a section in your salon procedures manual that clearly spells out how all checks are to be handled. Adequate procedures and safeguards will help reduce the problem of bounced checks. You will need to indicate what kinds of checks to accept or reject. Put samples of the checks in a training file for the staff to review. Ideally, you will have a receptionist or only one employee who handles all sales transactions, but if you don't, be sure everyone is adequately trained in this area.

Be cautious of

1. Two-party checks. These are written by a first party to a second party who endorses it so it can be cashed by a third party (you). These checks are susceptible to fraud because the first party can stop payment, leaving you without your funds.
2. Government checks. Be sure to know your endorser to make sure they were not stolen and the endorsement forged.
3. Traveler's checks. The main concern is to have them signed at the time they are presented for payment in the presence of the employee accepting them.
4. Checks written on nonlocal banks. Get both out-of-state and local addresses and telephone numbers on the back of the check.

Always notice the date on the check, and don't accept a check if the date is blank, post-dated, or over thirty days old. Checks should be made out for the service/purchase price only, not for cash over and above that amount. If the check bounces you could lose both, the cost of the service and the cash. And be sure to verify the person's identification, compare signatures, and make sure the check is payable to your salon.

You might want to have a policy of accepting only cash from new or nonregular customers until they become regular customers and you get to know them.

When a check is returned from your bank have the receptionist or whomever handles this activity log the customer name, address, and telephone number. Make several copies of the check and put the original in a safe place. Treat it as if it were cash.

Call the customer. Always be polite and give the customer the benefit of the doubt. Ask if you can redeposit the check. If the customer says yes, take it to the bank yourself. (I would suggest you first call the bank to make sure it will clear.) If the check still won't clear, call the customer again. Explain what the bank said and ask how you should handle this situation as quickly as possible. Depending on the answer and how he/she answers, proceed accordingly. Let the customer know your salon policy is to pursue this type of situation until it is resolved. You may want to work out a repayment schedule, plus interest and bank charges, if this seems to be the most desirable alternative. If you decide to use a collection agency, make sure the agency is a member in good standing of the American Collectors Association.

Be sure to maintain an adequate checking balance in your own business account to protect your normal operations. You do not want a balance so low that one or two returned checks from a customer will cause your business checks to bounce.

SMALL-CLAIMS COURT

The small-claims court is a relatively inexpensive and simple judicial forum for small civil disputes. For the particulars of the court in your area check with the courts clerk. This court is for civil, not criminal, disputes with a certain dollar limit. Some jurisdictions allow the use of juries, but this usually involves a fee. Juries are usually not advisable as the judges are capable, fair, and competent. In most states, the loser in the suit pays all court costs. Preparation is the key to success. Be able to prove every fact alleged in your claim.

The trial is fairly informal. Each party presents his or her own story and evidence and calls and questions witnesses. The judge may also question the witnesses and discuss the evidence.

To use this court, file your claim with the clerk of the court. Complete your name and address, the name and address of the party being sued (the defendant), indicate the amount of money for which you are suing, and the basis for your claim.

TURNING COMPLAINTS INTO SALES

There will always be some customers who would rather have a gripe than be satisfied. You should do everything possible to turn their complaints into sales. Develop empathy for the customer's plight; try to understand her feelings and the real problem. Listen attentively, and avoid getting defensive or angry. Concentrate on how you can solve the problem and provide satisfaction. Offer to redo the work, or replace the product if that is the problem, for free.

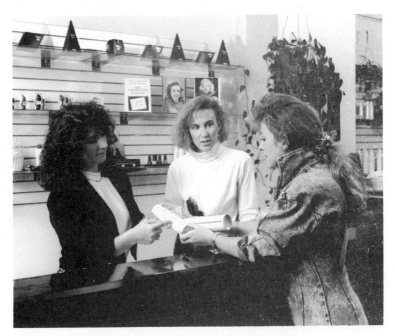

Always try to resolve complaints; don't evade or ignore them.

Always try to resolve complaints, don't evade or ignore them. An unhappy customer will remember the situation forever and will probably tell the story as often as possible—certainly more often than would be good for your business and professional reputation. It is simply good business sense to resolve customer complaints.

Finally, educate your customers. Some clients become unhappy about a service or product simply because they don't know what to expect or what it entails. Effective customer consultations can reduce customer complaints.

RESOLVING YOUR COMPLAINTS

If you are dissatisfied with a product or service, there are ways to get satisfaction. Take the item or issue up with the business involved, preferably the person with whom you originally dealt. If you don't get satisfaction, explain that you are prepared to pursue the matter. Get the person's name and the name and department of the person's supervisor.

Present your case to the manager, or next higher-up individual, in a clear, brief, factual manner without anger or threats. Explain why you think you deserve satisfaction. If you fail to get satisfaction, take the matter to the next higher level. Call the company to find out if there is a consumer affairs department or something similar. Be sure to get the name of the person you talk to and then again explain your situation/complaint.

If all else fails, ask for the name of the company president. Call or write the president, stating your problem and indicating who you talked to and when at the various company levels. If you call, make it person to person. Make sure you let the president know you expect action within a certain time frame.

Make sure you give your name, address, and telephone number. Let them know that you are sending copies of your complaint to the Better Business Bureau, your state's Consumer Protection Agency, the U.S. Office of Consumer Affairs in Washington, D.C., and to your state attorney general's office.

Make sure your letter goes by certified mail. If you still don't receive satisfaction, file your complaints. Demand a return for your time and trouble. Negotiate for the value of the time you have spent trying to resolve your problem. You must be aggressive and persevere if you are to receive satisfactory results.

Better Business Bureau

The Better Business Bureau (BBB) was formed to promote truth and accuracy in advertising. They also handle customer complaints, even though they are not an enforcement agency. The BBB is not a policing organization, and doesn't have any authority over individual businesses. It can expel members and can notify an inquirer if a business has a history of not resolving complaints.

The BBB is also devoted to education of its members on a wide range of topics and is designed as a self-regulating body for businesses. Membership is usually interpreted as supporting the ideals and functions of the organization and is a signal that a member supports the concept and ideals of better business for the general public.

Being a member of the BBB is a good way to meet other business owners and to make potentially good contacts that at some time or other may be of benefit to your business.

Chamber of Commerce

The chamber of commerce is designed more for the benefit of businesses. The goals of the chamber of commerce are to strengthen the economy, improve the quality of life, and represent business interests to all levels of government. They offer business assistance through seminars and clinics, which is of particular interest to small businesses. They also offer, in varying degrees, consulting services. The chamber of commerce makes available various resource publications, which could be very informative for you, that are specific to their regional location. It is also an alternate source of some insurance.

SUMMARY

Many things are involved in the day-to-day operations of a salon. To be successful you must be prepared to handle all issues that arise, including shipping, bounced checks, and customer complaints. You also must be able to resolve your own complaints and know where to go for assistance.

Managing a staff is a time-consuming and critical task. It is up to you to set the dress code for the salon and assure that all salon rules and regulations are followed. To keep employees motivated and performing up to your standards you must be aware of their needs and always communicate honestly with them. Regular staff meetings are essential, and all employees should be encouraged to participate in them.

Proper and continuing training is vital if you and your employees are to stay abreast of changes and developments in your field. Trade shows are excellent sources of information. Always keep them in mind when preparing your annual budget.

PERSONAL DEVELOPMENT

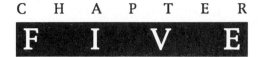

C H A P T E R

F I V E

As a salon owner, you will need to learn to be an effective manager and leader. There is much to be taken into consideration, including the ability to delegate tasks to employees, planning and organizing, problem solving, communication and listening skills, interpersonal skills, product knowledge, and of course, customer skills.

PERSONAL EVALUATION

You must do a personal evaluation to identify your weak points as a manager and leader. Then develop a personal development plan to become the best you can be.

Administrative Skills

This involves the ability to structure your own activities and the activities of your staff and the ability to utilize resources in a way that maximizes productivity and efficiency. This results in satisfaction to your customers and employees. Some administrative skills you should develop include delegation, expense control, group facilitation, follow through, planning, and time management.

1. Delegation. Define and assign tasks to employees to develop their commitment and competence.

2. Expense control. Monitor and control all expenses at realistic levels.
3. Group facilitation. Lead the staff to achieve objectives and develop teamwork; learn how to plan and conduct meetings.
4. Monitoring/follow through. Establish and utilize a procedure for regularly checking progress.
5. Planning and organizing skills. Establish priorities, anticipate problems, and determine realistic completion dates.
6. Time management. Establish priorities and use time effectively to meet commitments and keep promises.

Cognitive Skills

This is knowledge that comes through perception, reasoning, or intuition. You must use that knowledge to learn new materials, to identify and define problems, and to make decisions.

1. Analytical skills. Separate data and information into elemental parts and arrive at the appropriate conclusions; identify problems and opportunities effectively and efficiently.
2. Problem solving. Demonstrate a disciplined thought process to each situation, and seek out innovative alternatives prior to evaluating and making a decision. Anticipate problems and be prepared to propose solutions.

Communications Skills

Communication is the ability to receive and interpret information clearly, accurately, thoroughly, and effectively. To communicate well you must be able to give and receive feedback. You also need to develop good listening, presentation, and reading skills.

1. Giving feedback. Deliver timely information about a product and/or service and present this information in a constructive manner.
2. Receiving feedback. Hear others' responses and/or reactions to yourself without needing to explain or rationalize.
3. Listening skills. Understand what is being said. This involves encouraging dialogue with eye contact and expression to seek clarification and confirmation.
4. Presentation skills. Retain an audience's attention through verbal and nonverbal communication. Use visual aids to focus the staff's attention on primary points of the subject.

5. Reading skills. Understand the intent and identify important factors in written information.
6. Verbal communication. Express yourself effectively, clearly, and succinctly in one-on-one discussions and in groups. State facts in a logical order, respond to others in an easily understood manner, and speak when appropriate.
7. Written communication. Express thoughts clearly and effectively; use appropriate style, grammar, spelling, and tone in formal and informal business communications.

Customer Skills

You must establish and maintain understandings of the needs of your customers. Combine sensitivity to salon capabilities with commitment to customer service by delivering timely, quality, and value-added products and services. You should develop both your sales and your service skills.

1. Sales skills. Use consultative selling skills. Identify customers' needs and motivate customers to make a decision. Instill confidence by responding to customers in a prompt, courteous, and informative manner. Manage phone conversations and use customer service and interpersonal skills to extract information and to deal effectively with abrupt, upset, or angry individuals.
2. Service skills. Demonstrate knowledge of the customer and respond to the customer's needs.

Human Resource Skills

This involves the ability to match an individual's skills to a given position. To assist with development of employees to their full potential, to recognize and reward performance fairly and equitable, and to effectively communicate strengths as well as development needs.

1. Interviewing/selection. Use appropriate questioning techniques to effectively identify and match a candidate's knowledge, skills, abilities, and traits to your position requirements.
2. Compensation management. Reward and reinforce positive employee performance or behavior through the effective use of compensation programs such as merit/promotional increases, incentive pay, or special awards.

3. Performance appraisal. Plan, conduct, and follow through on performance appraisals. Constructively communicate with positive and negative information.

Interpersonal Skills

As a salon owner, you must have the ability to behave in a manner appropriate to the situation and to the individuals involved. You must understand and be sensitive to the behavior of others and handle conflicts positively. It is important for you to develop conflict resolution and negotiation skills.

1. Conflict resolution/confrontation skills. Recognize and use conflict as an opportunity for improved organizational and individual productivity. Create a win/win situation by using a joint problem solving approach to meet the needs of all parties.
2. Negotiation skills. Develop and use the strategies, tactics, and countermeasures required to conclude a win/win situation.
3. Persuasiveness. Sell your ideas and influence others.
4. Professionalism. Interact with others by demonstrating courtesy, honesty, respect, and competence; always be a positive role model.
5. Teamwork. Work cooperatively with salon staff and customers and integrate personal skills with those of others to accomplish the salon's goals. Keep personal interests subordinated to the overall salon objectives.

Job Knowledge

You should have a thorough understanding of the overall technical content, purpose, key responsibilities, and required results of each job in your salon.

1. Product knowledge. Recognize features and benefits of various products and maintain up-to-date and complete familiarity with the full range of products offered, including the features and benefits.
2. Technical knowledge. Comprehend the required information particular to a job or service offered.

Leadership Skills

Good leadership involves inspiring others to action by articulating a clear direction or vision. You can achieve a desired goal by directing the activities of others. Try to practice participative management and model the behaviors required for success. Select, train, develop, and motivate others and support a stable and open workplace.

1. Decisiveness. Arrive at final conclusions without unwarranted delay and communicate decisions in a confident manner.
2. Development skills. Plan for and implement activities with the staff so they can achieve personal and professional goals.
3. Direction/goal-setting skills. Establish realistic and challenging goals and plans and ensure that individual goals are compatible with the goals and priorities of the salon.
4. Managing diversity. Recognize, appreciate, and encourage viewpoints and values different from your own.
5. Motivating others. Create a work environment that inspires top performance and encourages the staff to share ideas and information openly. Always keep the salon staff well informed.
6. Teambuilding. Obtain satisfactory end results through group participation. Generate group interaction by soliciting ideas, opinions, and suggestions from all members of the salon staff, and provide an environment in which each staff member has the opportunity to contribute equally.
7. Training skills. Assist others to do their job and/or enhance their knowledge base.

You will probably find that most obstacles to management and leadership growth will be that your needs or weaknesses are simply not recognized. It is easy to convince yourself that you don't have enough time to devote to your personal development or that any change simply requires too much planning, thinking, and hard work. You can convince yourself that it is human nature to resist change. But if you need to improve yourself as a manager you must take the initiative to do so. No one else will do it for you; in fact, no one else will even care. It is your salon and your responsibility to make it succeed by being the very best manager you can be.

BE ASSERTIVE

Learning to be assertive can help improve the way you communicate with people. You must, especially as a business person, be in control or you will be controlled. Being assertive means learning how to say no when you should or when you have to, without the emotional drawbacks of feeling guilty, hurt, or angry. It means saying what is on your mind, honestly and directly but not with the intent of offending or hurting others. It is saying what you mean to say, saying what you think, asking for what you want, and refusing what you do not want.

If you are not an assertive person now, learning to become so will not change your personality or make you pushy or unpopular. It will improve your skills as a business professional, your feelings and attitudes about yourself, and perhaps even the quality of your life. You will gain respect for yourself and others will respect you also.

Learning to be assertive is easier for some than for others. But it can be done and it is important for you to develop this skill. You may have to attend a formal training session or complete a thorough self-study course to help you develop this skill but it is worth it. A book I would recommend is Jean Baer's *How to Be an Assertive (not aggressive) Woman in Life, in Love, and on the Job*. Read it and give yourself an edge over your competition.

SUMMARY

The success of your salon depends on you and your abilities. If you are not assertive enough or need to improve your leadership and management skills you must seek assistance. Recognize your weak points and work on improving them—no one else can do it for you.

To be an effective manager you must develop your administrative, communication, human resource, and interpersonal skills. You must have a thorough knowledge of all jobs performed in the salon and be adept at working with customers of all kinds.

BUSINESS DEVELOPMENT

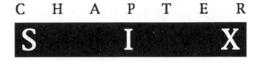

C H A P T E R
SIX

Customers come and go for any number of reasons. To keep up with rising expenses and to improve your overall profitability, you will always need to be actively involved in developing and recruiting new customers. This will continually be one of your top priorities. Even though you will have created the most attractive salon and hired and trained the best technicians, you cannot succeed without a steady flow of customers. In this chapter, you will learn different ways to attract new customers, as well as how to keep the ones you have, and what to do about customers who are consistently late or don't show up.

CULTIVATING CUSTOMERS

During your initial preplanning process, you identified your target clientele (the type of customers you want in your salon) and the services you wanted to offer. If you are just starting out you cannot count on word-of-mouth referrals and you shouldn't count on walk-ins or someone finding you by chance. You must take the initiative to actively cultivate new customers.

A simple truth is that the more contacts you make and the more people you tell about your salon, the more customers you will have. This will include friends and relatives, business professionals (they must have nice looking nails too), chance casual meetings (always carry business cards), and association prospecting. Keep a sharp eye open for anyone whose hands are highly visible and in need of your services, such as receptionists, waitresses, and professionals. You must constantly be on the lookout for opportunities to sell yourself and your salon.

Always remember to build your creditability with each and every customer. You and your technicians must know your business better than anyone else, dress appropriately, act and be professional and ethical at all times. You must know your customers and what type of products and services they want. You and your staff must treat each and every customer with respect and "pamper" them.

When explaining procedures and home maintenance programs to your customers, keep your dialogue simple and nontechnical. Don't confuse your customers but explain things patiently and simply. Sell concepts and benefits. Outline the pros and cons of various treatments or services and respectfully convince the customer as to the proper choices.

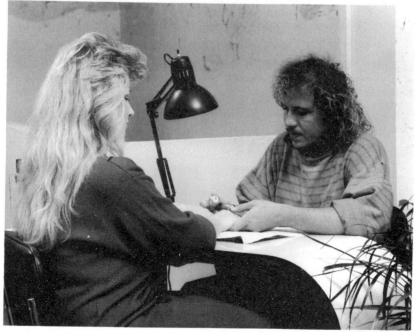

Outline the pros and cons of various treatments or services and respectfully convince the customer of the proper choices.

Always be enthusiastic and communicate in a positive, assertive manner. Make your customers glad they come to your salon for their nail care treatments.

First Impression

Create a good first impression for your salon by insisting on good telephone etiquette. That first impression is created when a customer calls your salon. Have the telephone answered as quickly as possible; don't let it ring. When using the telephone hold, have music to lessen the impact of waiting or a recorded message about your salon products and services. If a customer is put on hold, always handle the call again within sixty seconds.

Brochures

You will want to educate people as to why they should come to your salon. To help facilitate this you will want to have brochures printed that describe your salon products and services. You should also have educational brochures that cover common problems or concerns, such as tough nails or nail biters, and how your salon services address them.

Business Cards

Pass out business cards freely and often—they are one of your best forms of advertisement. When having your cards printed, don't skimp on the quality of the paper or printing. Make them impressive, yet simple and elegant.

Promotions

Hold business card drawings in the salon. Have customers leave their business cards for a drawing for a free manicure or service you wish to promote. This is a good source of company contacts. Call the company personnel department or employee relations department to get your advertising message in their company newsletter. Personally visit each company once a contact has been established to find out what opportunities may exist for you. Many companies have benefits throughout the year where they auction off products or services to raise money. Donate some of your gift certificates that can be auctioned off in order to receive good publicity for your salon.

Ask your customers to collect and deposit their friends' business cards for a drawing where they both can win. Simply have the

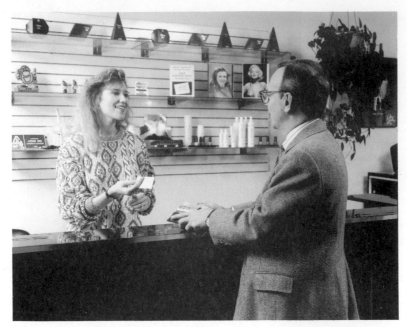

Pass out business cards freely and often.

customer write their name on the back of their friend's business card for your drawing.

Offer current customers a free service for every five new customers they refer to your salon. Have a two-for-one offer—if the customer brings a friend they both get a service for the price of one.

Look for opportunities to demonstrate your products and services such as at theme shows at shopping malls, schools, or fairs. If tourism is big in your area, contact the local hotels, motels, and inns to see if you can leave your business cards and/or brochures in their guest rooms.

Holidays

Holidays present both opportunities and problems that must be recognized and planned for. Count on frantic schedules caused by last-minute cancellations, late clients, emergency repairs, last-minute requests for nail care, walk-ins, and who knows what else. After you have been in business for a while, review and analyze your prior years' schedules and results. Identify your busy days and hours. Hire additional staff; start early to interview, hire, and train. You might hire extra staff to handle just certain tasks, such as manicuring, walk-ins, or emergencies.

Encourage your regular customers to book as far ahead as possible. Be sure to call each customer the day before to confirm all appointments. Keep a waiting list of new clients or last-minute requests so as to fit them into any cancellation. Schedule appointments so that you can allow a little extra time for the technician to catch her breath and relax so the heavy schedule will be less stressful.

Maintain quality standards even through a hectic schedule. Be sure to continue to pamper and give each client the attention each deserves.

Avoid running out of supplies and products during the holiday seasons. Be sure to order ahead of time everything you will need to handle a business volume of up to 25 percent more than your usual monthly needs. December is by far the busiest month of the year and you certainly do not want to run out of anything, particularly products the technicians use on clients.

You are responsible for defining specific objectives and direction, then deciding which promotions will accomplish your objectives. Early planning is essential and is your responsibility. Remember, in addition to maintaining superior quality service through the hectic and demanding holiday seasons, service or product promotions will:

1. Bring in extra income for the salon and staff.
2. Help you show appreciation to your clientele.
3. Improve public relations.
4. Give you a good fast start for January business.
5. Possibly become a tradition with the salon.

GREETINGS Send holiday greetings to your clients. The time and expense is well worth the goodwill your salon will receive. One note of caution: Select a greeting that will not offend anyone's religious preference or beliefs.

ADVERTISING Plan your advertising early and double-check the due dates so as not to miss any important publications. Set up a calendar so you won't slip up. Holiday seasons are too important to miss.

DECORATING   Salon decorating is very important during the holiday seasons for your clientele and for your staff. It's particularly good for staff morale. Encourage everyone to participate in the spirit of the season.

GIFT CERTIFICATES   Gift certificates are important at all times but are especially important during holidays and particularly so at Christmas. Be sure to have plenty on hand. As a special promotion, if a customer buys two for a friend or relative, give the customer a discount on her next visit. Be sure to let your clients know you have gift certificates with an obvious but appropriate display. Encourage the salon staff to mention gift certificates to their customers. You might even offer a prize or bonus to whomever sells the most gift certificates. Be creative and innovative.

Important Holiday Reminders

- Make sure your advertising meets the various deadline dates for whatever medium you choose.
- Plan early for sufficient inventories of supplies, products, retail items, and accessories. (Plan on doubling your normal usage.)
- Be sure to adjust staff working hours to handle the increased workload.
- A procedure must be in place to call clients one to two days prior to their appointment to confirm the day and time. You cannot afford unplanned cancellations.
- Establish a waiting list so as to fill any cancellations that do occur.
- Establish a procedure to follow-up with new clients who visited the salon during the holiday season. You don't want to lose them.
- Remind all clients to book early. Appointments will be hard to get and you will want your regular customers to have priority.
- Record all gifts from customers so you can send a thank-you note.

FOCUS GROUPS

Focus groups are used to develop an honest, useful consensus of opinions and suggestions that can be incorporated into your salon operations to improve your success and to capitalize on your salon's strengths. Such feedback also helps to get a clearer view of your clients' wants, needs, likes, and dislikes. This helps you to identify what keeps them happy and coming back instead of going to another salon.

Select a number of regular customers whose opinions you respect and who are articulate and willing to share their opinions. Also include a number of infrequent customers for balance and perspective. You will want a group of approximately ten individuals, one that isn't so large it would impede active participation by any one member. You might want to structure your guidelines so as to have new customers rotate into the group as you rotate others out so that no one individual participates longer than twelve months.

As with all other aspects of your business to achieve success and beneficial results that would justify your time and effort, you must plan how you will conduct your meeting. Work out all the details, procedures, and objectives for the group. If you have not had experience or training as a group facilitator, I would recommend you either study the techniques required or plan on having your meetings chaired by a trained interviewer/facilitator to avoid personality pitfalls and to keep the meeting moving along according to the agenda. You want your meeting to be positive and constructive instead of being a social gathering.

At your initial meeting you will want to review the purpose of the meeting and what you wish to achieve. You will want to encourage everyone to be open, honest, fair, and participative. You will want to avoid wasting anyone's time and acquiring useless information and feedback. You will need to be very specific as to what kind of feedback you want.

Follow these guidelines when preparing your list of queries for your focus group.

1. Focus on important issues and ask only necessary questions.
2. Be very clear with your questions and queries. Avoid technical terms, industry jargon, and ambiguous words.
3. Encourage specific responses instead of generalizations.
4. Avoid asking leading questions or wording questions to encourage a specific or suggested response. You want honest feedback that you can use, not information you would like to hear.

5. Keep questions simple and address one point at a time. Don't ask for several pieces of information in the same question.
6. The sequence of your questions is important. Ask interesting questions first, difficult questions in the middle, and the least important questions last.

Be sure to hold your meetings in private, such as in a separate dining room at a restaurant or at the salon when it is closed. Lunch is usually an ideal time for such a group meeting. Of course the salon picks up the check if the meeting is held at a restaurant or provides snacks and refreshments if the meeting is held in the salon.

EDUCATING THE CUSTOMER

Your technicians have a responsibility to your salon and customers, but your customers also have a responsibility—to take proper care of their nails. What's the solution to help educate your customers? In addition to verbal instructions by the technician, which may or may not be completely understood, you should utilize a customer information card or pamphlets. You can include information on sculptured nails, natural nails, basic foot care, and general salon services.

Use only one topic per card or pamphlet. When designing your cards or pamphlets be sure to make them elegant. They should be printed on good quality paper with your salon logo, address, telephone number, and a space for the technician's name. Make your information cards or pamphlets as professional as your salon.

You should also have cards made for your salon use—for a release agreement, a customer history, or any other purpose you may want.

Customer Release Agreement

A customer release agreement is a form the customer signs allowing you to do nail work that is against your better judgment. For example, you have a customer with a problem nail that you feel should be treated by a physician, but for whatever reason the customer insists that you do what you can. If the situation is somewhat borderline, and not an obvious emergency or serious situation, you may choose to do the work. However, your release agreement should clearly state the condition of the nail, that you did not want to do the work, that you recommended the problem be treated by a physician, and that you agreed to do the work only if you would be held completely harmless from any responsibility in case the problem deteriorated. Have the customer date and sign the agreement.

Do not give anyone else in the salon the authority to use these release agreements. You are getting into potentially serious situations and you alone should make this decision. Have your attorney prepare your release agreement so you will be as well protected as possible.

The release agreement should also have space for information on the results of a patch test, information on any allergies, special medication, and the client's doctor's name.

Having said that, in my opinion it is always better not to do any nail work against your better judgment and especially if you believe it is actually wrong to do it. Sometimes it is better to have an angry customer than risk legal trouble or harming someone. I don't mean to belabor this point because in my experience it is relatively infrequent, but it is better to be prepared for any situation. When it comes to health issues, it is always better to error on the side of caution.

Personal History Card

You need to spend time with each new client so you can determine what treatment the customer needs, what you will do, how the treatment will benefit the customer and what the customer can expect. This initial "getting acquainted" period is very important and can go a long way to impress upon the client your professionalism and to start the process of maintaining a long-term relationship with the client. This session should be recorded on a customer personal history card.

A personal history card should include the name of the customer, address, work and home telephone numbers, space for each date of service, remarks about any problems or conditions of the nails so that anyone who may serve the customer will know the history.

Preventing No-Shows

Customers who make appointments and fail to keep them without calling to cancel are a major problem for technicians and salon owners. It means lost income to the technician and the salon. There are any number of reasons why people don't keep appointments. Perhaps the customer cannot locate the salon or is unsure of your work quality.

The customer may decide at the last minute that her nails can wait, or maybe she heard "horror stories" about having nails done, such as exaggerations about fungus or damaged nails.

For first-time customers, nails are usually an "impulse" decision, which means the service should be provided as quickly as possible. Try to get the person into the salon within forty-eight hours of making the appointment. If the appointment is for a full set of nails and you can't do the work within this time frame, at least get the customer in for a free sample nail to demonstrate your skill. This works in many instances to save a new customer and will address most of the concerns a new customer may have. It also gives you an opportunity to address those concerns and to create a favorable impression.

Fill In Those Cancellations

Cancellations do happen and in most cases for legitimate reasons. However, if you educate your customers so as to get them to call in advance to cancel, your loss can be minimized. You can fill the cancellation time slot with someone else. Time is money, so don't waste it.

The receptionist, or someone else if you don't have a receptionist, should keep a waiting list of customers who want to come in for appointments. The list should contain the client's name, home and work telephone numbers, and the nail work or service that is requested.

WEDDINGS

Over five million women get married every year. This number of brides, plus the wedding party, equates to a lot of potential new customers for everyone. And even the men in the wedding parties are potential customers. How many weddings occur each year in your area?

While people marry throughout the year, Christmas and Valentine's Day are the largest engagement seasons that start brides thinking about plans for their weddings. June through September have the most actual number of weddings. You want to get as much of this market as you can.

Attend bridal fairs and shows and distribute professionally printed leaflets that promote your special packages for brides and their wedding parties. Try to get the fairs' promoters to provide you with the names and addresses of everyone who attends for use with your follow-up mail campaign.

You can even participate in a show or fair by buying booth space. This can be a good idea, but check the costs and benefits to you very carefully. Exactly what will it cost you? How many new customers would you have to attract to cover this expense? Can your salon handle this additional workload? Do some research on the producers of the show. Check their credentials and references, and evaluate their track record. Also consider:

- What is the number of attendees from prior shows?
- What are the demographics of the show's attendees? Are these the type of potential customers that would visit your salon?
- Who will the other exhibitors be? Will there be an adequate number to attract a large attendance? Are they professional?
- What is the timing of the show? Will it catch the local wedding season? Will it conflict with major holidays or with other popular local events?

You might want to donate nail services to the models at the bridal fashion shows in exchange for signage, giving your salon credit for the nail work. And you should offer wedding party group discounts.

Other sources include:

1. Contact the bridal consultants listed in the yellow pages. They are often asked to refer a nail salon.
2. Try to get bridal shops to let you put your business cards on display for their customers. Establish a referral relationship with the bridal shops—something like a gift certificate from your salon if a customer buys a wedding dress. Make friends with the clerks and salespeople, and occasionally give them a free manicure.
3. Make contacts with wedding photographers. They are also a potential source of referrals.
4. Contact your local jewelers and offer to sell them your gift certificates. The jewelers give their customers the gift certificate with the purchase of a ring.

5. Newspapers usually have special bridal issues around spring time. This is a good place to advertise.
6. Radio and television sales representatives often know about local bridal promotions.

Depending on the size of your salon staff, you may be able to do the whole wedding party at the same time. If so, set aside the appropriate time and provide refreshments. Be sure to encourage members of the bridal party to book their appointments in advance to avoid last-minute problems. Encourage the bride to come in at least two weeks early in order to get used to nails and to have time for repair and a maintenance session before the big wedding day.

With the attention hands get at weddings and receptions, the groom's nails are also a target of opportunity for you.

SENIOR CITIZENS

Senior citizens are the fastest growing segment of our population, with women making up the majority of this group. Appearance is important at any age, but especially for women getting older. As a rule, women take more pride in their appearance when they are older than when they were younger. Most older women identify themselves as being five to ten years younger than their actual age. Keep this in mind when servicing them.

It is most important to remember that an older woman doesn't see herself as old as you see her. Give her the same options you would give a younger woman. Don't generalize or make assumptions about physical restrictions, as physical ailments can occur at any age.

Never shout or raise your voice at an older person, especially during initial greetings. Many older people who are hard of hearing are sensitive to facial expressions and mannerisms and someone shouting often looks upset to them. If in doubt, ask if she can hear you. Trust your judgment. Avoid walking in front of an older person, as she may need to pace herself and gauge her steps in advance. You don't want to cause any inconvenience.

Comfort, especially as regards manicure chairs, is more important for the older customers than it is for your younger customers. Lighting is also very important. If you have overhead lights, use them. The normal aging eyes need three times as much light as younger eyes. Be sure to listen carefully to older clients and be patient. Senior citizens do make an excellent customer segment so don't dismiss them lightly. Make your salon a meeting place and socializing place for the older customer and increase your volume of business.

KEEPING THAT CLIENT

Now that you have the customer in your salon your next objective is to keep the person coming back. Keeping your current customers is far less expensive than continually having to find new ones. You can be a good technician with good skills, but if your attitude, appearance, or actions do not convey professionalism, you will lose the customer to another salon.

Attitude

Attitude is important and definitely will affect your ability to attract and retain clients, and in fact affect every facet of your professional and personal life. Work on being positive by focusing on what is good and right instead of on negatives. Focus on the positive qualities of people and circumstances around you. Build a cooperative, participative, energetic, and dynamic team spirit within the salon. Be service oriented. Remember, having nails done is a luxury so for people to come to your salon to spend their money there must be adequate incentives. They must receive good quality for their money and friendly, superior service. Strive to develop a happy, friendly staff. Always work to improve your own and your staff's interpersonal skills, and always practice self-control. Don't get involved in pettiness or with people with negative attitudes.

As an owner, your commitment to proper attitudes goes even further. You must observe all government regulations dealing with employees, such as minimum wages. You certainly don't ever want to give the impression of cheating anyone—employees, customers, or suppliers. You shouldn't attempt to "steal" employees from other salons. Always be sensitive to setting a good example and to maintaining an atmosphere in the salon that encourages ethical behavior.

Foster respect for all clients and treat each and every one as the most important person in your salon. Even difficult customers must be treated fairly and with a smile. Technicians must be punctual for their appointments, keep their stations clean and neat, avoid smoking and eating at their stations, and not be allowed to accept personal telephone calls when with a customer. Every customer should receive better service than expected.

Finally, don't condone, encourage, or participate in gossip. Nothing good comes from gossip. If it starts, change the subject at the first polite opportunity. Keep discussions on the client's nails or on a noncontroversial topic. Don't gossip about other salons. Remember to continually remind your staff that if you can't say something nice about someone or something, don't say anything. Technicians should never talk about:

Their salary/income
Their personal life
Personal financial problems
Salon management
Controversial subjects
Other salons' work or their employees
Other customers
Coworkers

Technicians should never argue with a customer, tell off-color jokes or use foul language, violate a confidence, or lose their temper.

Appearance

Appearance is as important as attitude. Your appearance is your best advertisement and will be critical to the success of you and your salon. This goes beyond wearing attractive nails and includes hairstyle; a clean, neat wardrobe; and proper use of cosmetics and fragrances. Look professional at all times.

Actions

The quality of work and service must be stressed and maintained at all times. Avoid having technicians too rushed for adequate time with customers. A realistic booking schedule is simply a matter of good business sense. Inconsistent training of new employees or a lack of appreciation for quality work must be avoided and corrected when it slips.

Personal attention to customers is the bedrock of customer relations. Always be willing to give extra of whatever is expected. You have spent too much time and effort to attract customers to have them leave your salon if you can prevent it. Most people feel that superior service is a little more important than price or convenience. Your salon must always be above your competition when it comes to service. If not, you will lose your customers.

Create an information card on each customer. Update this information card immediately after each customer visit, not at the end of the day or some other time when pertinent information may be forgotten. Include a section for:

- Name.
- Address.
- Telephone.
- Birthday.
- Interests/hobbies.
- Subjects to avoid.
- Latest personal happenings, such as promotions, a sick child, or wedding.
- Service history. (Include date, service, nail shape, polish color used, cost, and comments.)

Practice giving your regular customers the VIP treatment. Book them as far ahead of time as their schedule will allow, such as three or four months ahead. Create a waiting list of clients who want to be booked for each technician. Always call to verify the appointments the day before. A note of caution: Don't leave a message with family members because they, particularly a husband, may not know that your customer has her nails done.

WALK-INS

Walk-in or unexpected clients are both good and bad news. You always want new customers, but sometimes you have trouble working them into a tight schedule. If the individual is a regular customer definitely try to fit her in. If you can't, take her name and telephone number and call her at the first opportunity.

If the problem of walk-ins becomes too frequent you might have to schedule extra working hours at the end of the day or hire another technician. Don't treat walk-in clients too lightly; they can become good long-term customers.

SLOW SUMMERS

Business will normally slow down during the summer months because of vacations and people working in their gardens. With school out this is when most people with school age children travel. You can usually count on business being down 10 to 20 percent, depending on the demographics of your customer base.

However, there are activities you can do to minimize the impact of the summer months:

- Encourage your own staff to take their vacations during this time instead of the traditional holiday seasons, such as Christmas.
- Actively go after new business. Offer innovative promotions and specials to attract old and new customers.
- Promote pedicures especially hard during this time of year. With more people going to the beach and wearing sandals and leisure clothes this is a natural service for additional income.
- Offer a pedicure-manicure special with discounts when purchased together as a package.
- Offer a special on nail art for toes to match that of the finger-nails.
- Offer a summer polish clearance sale—buy-one-get-one-free or something similar.
- Develop a mailing list of newcomers to your area. Check with the telephone company, utility company, realtors, and county clerk for addresses. Send them an invitation to visit your salon and make an appointment. Personally follow-up to reinforce the contact and the appointment.

PUBLIC SPEAKING

The more successful you become and the more active you are in the community, the more opportunity you will have to speak or make presentations before groups of people. As you build your business you should seek out opportunities to address groups in order to promote your salon. This is free exposure and easier than you think. You may have to make the first move to line up your initial speaking engagement. Once you do, other groups will probably call you. This makes it important that you select the initial group to contact very carefully. If you don't know such a group to contact, a good source for information will be your own customers. Find out which groups they belong to and then express an interest in speaking to them. Consider the Rotary, ladies clubs, church groups, school groups, and garden clubs. Don't turn down opportunities and let your competition get ahead of you. When speaking, there are some common sense guidelines to follow:

1. Develop an easy, open facial expression to create a friendly reception with the group you are addressing. Smile and have fun.
2. To gain immediate attention, begin with a story, a question, or humor.
3. Use body language, in moderation, to emphasize your words.
4. At appropriate moments during your presentation, back up your facts with stories or examples.
5. Pause often to allow time to breath and to alleviate stress and before and after important points.
6. Maintain eye contact with your audience.
7. Keep your talk short and simple.
8. Communicate ideas, not just words.
9. End your presentation with a quote, a question, or a story, or leave them laughing.

On the other hand, there are practices you want to avoid:

1. Avoid being ill prepared. Practice your speech out loud using a tape recorder and a mirror.
2. Don't be long-winded and think that more is better.
3. Avoid being a note-reader with your eyes glued to your notes.
4. Avoid an inordinate amount of numbers or statistics.
5. Avoid speaking specifically and blatantly about your personal salon. Stick to generic subjects, such as the nail business, benefits of artificial nails, or natural hand care. Occasional examples of

your own personal experiences and situation to support or emphasize a point is certainly acceptable.

6. Don't write out a whole speech and try to memorize it. Instead, write in large capital letters on index cards the points to cover. Then practice your talk in front of a mirror as many times as it takes to become comfortable.

7. Avoid drinking and smoking until after you leave. Today, too many people may be offended so it isn't worth the risk.

Local groups will not expect a professional speaker so don't think you have to be one. They will prefer someone who is natural and local.

Prior to your speaking date, find out the number of people who will attend, their age groups, if the group will be men or women, and if you will be a solo speaker or part of a panel. Find out at what point in the meeting you will speak, how long you should speak, and if you should do any demonstrations or use visual aids. Also, find out if you can distribute business cards and/or literature on your salon.

SUMMARY

Customers are the reason your salon exists. Attracting new customers and keeping old ones should be your top priorities. Always provide the best service possible to assure that your customers will return and that they will recommend your salon to their friends.

Always be looking for new ways to attract customers. Participate in bridal shows and fairs, cultivate elderly clients, run special promotions, and take advantage of any opportunity to speak in public. Holidays could be your busiest times. Plan ahead to assure you do not run out of supplies or miss advertising deadlines.

Focus groups can be a good way to get feedback about your salon's operations and services. The group should contain approximately ten people and meet on a regular basis.

HEALTH AND SAFETY

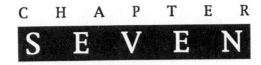
Insuring the protection of your employees and your customers is crucial when running a nail salon. You need to keep up your first aid knowledge and promote safety in your salon. In addition, you need to stay educated on many subjects, including AIDS, in order to ensure the safest environment.

SALON SAFETY

Salon safety, for your employees and customers, will be your responsibility as the owner of the salon. This goes above and beyond your insurance requirements. The following outline lists some ideas to keep in mind:

A. Telephone numbers
   1. Post all emergency telephone numbers in a conspicuous place, within easy access of a telephone.
B. Parking
   1. Make sure the parking area is well lit at all times. Any burned out light bulbs should be replaced as soon as possible.
   2. After dark, encourage a "buddy system" for customers and employees going to their parked cars. Have two individuals

walk together or at least have one person watch for the other one. When approaching parked automobiles:

a) Approach with caution.

b) Have the key out and ready to use.

c) Always check the back seat area and possibly even under the car.

d) Quickly get in and lock all doors.

C. Routine

1. Vary your routine of going to and from the salon. Walk a different route from time to time and park in different areas.

D. Cash

1. Don't keep a large amount of cash in the cash register, especially large bills. Use a safe for overflow receipts. Make frequent bank deposits and vary your deposit routine and schedule.

2. Be aware of counterfeit bills. Avoid accepting large bills unless the service amount justifies it.

E. Checks

1. For checks, have employees write "for deposit only" (or use a stamp) on the back of the check as soon as it is presented.

F. Credit Cards

1. Tear up or give the customer the credit card carbons.

G. Crime

1. Become friendly with your local police officers. Let them know of any unusual hours or if you will be transporting a large amount of cash. Solicit their advice on how you can better protect your salon.

2. Keep the salon well lit.

3. Have a safe place to store employee handbags. They should be out of sight and locked if possible. Also, if possible, change procedures and locations periodically.

H. Children

1. It is best to keep children out of the salon altogether. If this is to be your salon policy put up a sign that says because of insurance concerns you cannot allow children who are not receiving services in the salon.

2. Provide a restricted playing area with coloring books, toys, and play items.

3. Don't let children wonder around the salon.

The holiday season will present different safety situations in addition to the usual ones:

- Don't cover the windows completely with decorations. It is better to have a trim of some sort around the edges in order to leave a clear view into and out of the salon.
- Provide a safe place for customer handbags and holiday gift purchases.
- Don't put a Christmas tree in front of the window to block the view or near where smokers sit. A dry tree catches fire quickly and disaster can occur very quickly if someone is careless. Keep children away from the tree at all times.
- Take all safety precautions and complete your preparations early.

Review with your employees salon procedures for various instances that may come up, such as what to do if a robber came into the salon, if there was a fire, or if someone is caught shoplifting. Have a plan of action for each potential situation.

One final thought: Keep the salon doors locked after sunset and only admit individuals with an appointment. I am not attempting to be overreactive, but safety is a serious issue. You simply must plan and take every precaution that a prudent person would take.

First Aid

Be sure to have as part of your salon procedures manual a section on salon first aid. Plan how you want a medical emergency handled.

All appropriate emergency telephone numbers (emergency rooms, police, poison control center, paramedics) should be posted. Ideally they should be on a single card, laminated for protection, near a telephone. Be sure to keep these numbers updated. If necessary you can use "911," which is available in most areas. This will immediately connect you with the police and fire departments and flash your telephone number and address on a screen for their use.

You should check all chemical and product containers in your storage area regularly for leakage and seal and cap tightness. Make sure every product is labeled correctly, and dispose of any product that is questionable. Don't take any chances. Establish standards and procedures for use of products and chemicals at the workstations. You should also prepare a book listing, in alphabetical order, the chemicals you have in the salon. Indicate how each should be treated and, in particular, the antidote for each.

Periodically put on your "safety hat" and tour your salon for situations that could cause an accident. Look for torn or loose carpet, broken chairs, and defective equipment. Most insurance companies have a safety department that will inspect your premises and offer advice free of charge.

You should have a well-stocked first aid kit in the salon. Check it often and replace items that have been used. (It would be ideal to have someone trained in first aid procedures and CPR.) Have a fire extinguisher in the salon, and check it regularly. Make sure it is the right type of extinguisher for your particular needs. You can ask your fire department for their advice.

If you allow children in the salon, you should have a designated area for them. Most items in a salon could be described as an "attractive nuisance" to a child and many could be quite dangerous.

ALLERGIC REACTIONS

Because of the different products and chemicals in a salon and the large number of customers, there is the possibility that someone may experience an allergic reaction. This is another reason for accumulating pertinent information about all new clients and updating records from time to time.

You should always ask whether a customer has ever had a problem with nail services in the past. For new clients, or if a question arises, test the product on a single nail for possible reactions. Look for an immediate reaction, then wait twenty-four hours for a delayed reaction. If none develops, proceed with booking the service. If a reaction does occur, suggest the client consult a physician. Do not attempt to treat any symptoms. Mark the client's record so as to avoid using the product, and products with similar ingredients, on the client in the future.

CHEMICALS

According to the Hazard Evaluation System and Information Service of the California Occupational Health Program "most chemicals found in artificial nail products have not been adequately tested to find out whether they could harm a developing baby or affect the fertility of either men or women. The little information that is available is largely based on studies of test animals. There is almost no information from studies on humans."

Employers are required, by OSHA, to educate their employees about the chemicals they work with. You must make available to the employees Material Safety Data Sheets (MSDSs) on every product used in the salon. You must also effectively and routinely train your employees in the safe use of chemicals. You can get copies of MSDSs from the manufacturer or distributor of your products. As an additional safety precaution, take the MSDSs to your doctor for guidance as to any chemicals you should avoid having in your salon. If there are any, discuss them with the distributor so you can substitute other safer products.

Proper salon ventilation is very important for the safety of your employees and customers. Ideally, the work areas should have an even flow of fresh air with contaminated air drawn away before it is breathed.

Your salon procedures manual should specifically address your policies toward:

Storage of chemicals
Use of rubber gloves
Washing of hands with soap and water
Proper storage of food away from chemicals
No eating or drinking at workstations.

AIDS

AIDS stands for acquired immunodeficiency syndrome. It is a serious illness that harms the body's ability to fight infection. It is caused by the human immunodeficiency virus (HIV)—the AIDS virus. The AIDS virus may live in the human body for years before actual symptoms appear. During the incubation period there may be no sign that a person is infected with HIV. However, the person can still pass the virus on to others. As the infection progresses, people may notice severe and lasting symptoms, including:

- Swollen lymph glands in the neck, underarm, or groin area
- Recurrent fever, including "night sweats"
- Rapid weight loss for no apparent reason
- Constant tiredness
- Diarrhea and decreased appetite
- White spots or unusual blemishes in the mouth.

Most people infected with HIV go on to develop AIDS. Their immune system becomes severely weakened, turning normally mild or rare diseases into potentially fatal conditions. One common illness of this type is *Pneumocystis carinii* pneumonia, an infection of the lungs. This illness is highly uncommon among healthy individuals. HIV may also attack the nervous system, causing damage to the brain and spinal cord.

An employee or client on whom AIDS-contaminated nippers, scissors, or other instruments are used is at risk if the instrument draws blood. However, the chance of anyone becoming infected in this manner is considered to be very small. AIDS is hard to get, and you can't get it through normal everyday contact—in a swimming pool; from mosquito bites, sweat, tears, clothes, or a telephone; by riding on a bus; or from sharing eating utensils or a drinking glass.

AIDS is getting more attention and concern today and rightly so. There is growing concern in the workplace that you will have to address. At some time you may have to deal with an employee or customer with the AIDS virus. You must develop an AIDS policy for your salon and put it in writing in your salon procedures manual. Be sure to check with your attorney to learn about your rights and those of your customers. Don't discriminate. You will be legally bound to apply your written salon policies without exception. You must be consistent in their application.

To the best of my knowledge, there has not been a reported case of AIDS being contacted during normal nail salon services. But a risk of transmission exists if instruments come in contact with contaminated blood. Even though experts say that a situation conducive to the transmission of AIDS in the nail salon is extremely rare, you should establish certain salon standards (again, check with your attorney and doctor for guidance). Technicians should avoid direct contact with open sores, abrasions, and cuts. They should also wear disposable gloves or at least have all cuts and abrasions covered with bandages.

Refer to OSHA Instruction CPL 2-2.44B regarding AIDS (HIV-1), hepatitis b (HBV) and hospital grade tuberculocidal disinfectants.

New techniques and procedures are being developed and updated at an accelerating pace, so check with your doctor for the latest sterilization techniques and products. Always keep abreast of the latest techniques, procedures, and information. For additional information about AIDS call the U.S. Public Health Service hotline (1-800-342-AIDS) or the National AIDS Information Clearinghouse (1-800-458-5231).

SUMMARY

The safety of your salon is crucial to its success. Always be aware of health and safety issues for the protection of your employees and customers as well as for yourself. Plan and prepare for every situation that could come up.

Do all you possibly can to protect your salon against crime. Be especially careful around holidays when crime rates rise and salon decorations could create additional safety hazards. Develop a policy regarding children in the salon and post it.

First aid procedures should be addressed in your procedures manual. Be sure to post all emergency telephone numbers and keep a well-stocked first aid kit on the premises. Chemicals used in the nail industry can be dangerous. Review all MSDSs carefully and cover all policies regarding the use and storage of chemicals in your procedure manual. Your procedures manual should also address the issue of AIDS.

SERVICES

C H A P T E R
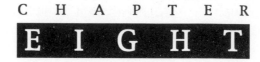
E I G H T

Now we get to the reasons for which customers come to your salon—to be pampered, to be cheered up, and to look and feel better when they leave than they did when they arrived. Previously I've made reference to different types of services you may want to offer to make your customers feel pampered and beautiful. Now it's time to get more specific.

As mentioned earlier, I feel the more services you offer the more profitable and interesting your salon will be. There is nothing wrong with one-stop shopping for personal beauty. It is easy to justify providing more than one or two services. Who would want to send a customer elsewhere to spend their beauty dollars?

SCHEDULING

Before we get into specific services, remember that you need to be as aware of your clients' busy schedules as your own. Time is critical, both to you and to the majority of your customers. When scheduling services, allow more time for new or nonregular clients. Give yourself plenty of time for the service, plus enough time to clean and set up the work area for the next customer. Outstanding service is critical to your success. Today's clientele expects better service than ever before and is willing to pay for it. Customers will know when service is not satisfactory. If you don't provide it, someone else will. Plan on being the best.

Initial Consultation

For new customers, the owner or manager should complete an initial consultation/evaluation before any treatment is started. Always be fair and honest with the customer. If a procedure should not be done because of medical concerns, refer the customer to a physician. If there is no reason not to proceed with what the customer wants, explain in detail what you think should be done and how you recommend the service should be provided.

Examine the nail carefully. Pay particular attention to the color of the nail bed. The pinker the nail bed, the healthier the nail and the better the circulation. Note any discoloration, inflammation, swelling, deformities, or nail separation from the nail bed. Analyze the nail flexibility and its thinness, thickness, texture, and roughness. Inquire about present nail care. Also inquire about the customer's current lifestyle and hobbies so as to better understand what kind of service to offer. Put all this information on a customer card for future reference. Update the information immediately after each visit.

MANICURES

Manicures, if done properly and in a timely manner, are probably more profitable than any service you can offer. A manicure is ideal for customers without artificial nails but who want natural nail care, which is a newer and growing trend. Manicures are an excellent service for women and men. A full range of manicures can also attract potential artificial nail customers to your salon. Failure to offer manicures will cause you to lose a good group of regular, profitable customers. I would strongly recommend that you perfect a variety of manicure techniques and services with a range of fees for each. Also, combine a manicure with a pedicure, waxing, or nail art to increase your sales even further.

Hot Oil Manicure

A hot oil manicure is simply a basic manicure, but electric mittens are used for about ten minutes followed by a warm lotion massage of the hands, wrists, and forearms. This is an excellent, popular, and profitable service.

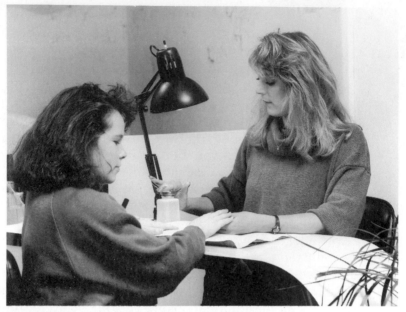

Manicures, if done properly and in a timely manner, are probably more profitable than any service you can offer.

WRAPS

Wraps were developed hundreds of years ago as a method of repairing damaged or torn nails. Wraps are used to repair or correct split, cracked, or damaged nails; to give added strength to short, weak nails; and/or to protect long nails from damage.

Wraps are thin, so as the nail grows there is not a ridge as with acrylics. Applying a wrap is easier than most people imagine. As with anything though, patience and practice is required to become proficient. Always caution your technicians to concentrate on the quality of the service rather than speed.

Following are some helpful hints in products.

1. Never try an unlabeled fabric on a client before testing adhesive compatibility.
2. Stick with products that are marketed specifically for the nail industry. These products have been tested and generally provide

the tightness and evenness of the weave the nail technician requires.

3. Read the manufacturer's instructions carefully. Many have 800-numbers for information and clarification of instructions.

4. Avoid mixing and matching products from different manufacturers unless you thoroughly check out each item. If you want to use a product from Company A with Company B's system, call Company B to verify that it will work and not create a problem.

5. Some clients may be sensitive to some of the products used. Do a patch test or test a nail before doing a full set of wraps.

6. Always keep an adequate inventory of adhesive, wrap material, files, buffers, alcohol, etc. to avoid having to turn away a customer.

There are many variations of the techniques for applying wraps. Check the instructions for the individual products you choose to use. With experience, you will develop your own method of application.

Types of Wraps

For many years wraps were made out of every type of cloth imaginable. Today, wraps come in four basic types: paper, silk, linen, and fiberglass. For each type there are treated or untreated wraps. An untreated wrap is plain and unadulterated (no glue). It is fairly economical, absorbs glue well, is less likely to lift (if applied properly), and will require a little more skill to apply than a treated wrap.

Treated wraps have adhesive on the back for easier application. No glue is required for the wrap to stick to the nail. There is, however, an increased chance of lifting so a top layer of glue should be applied when the wrap is put on the nail. Treated wraps naturally cost a little more than untreated wraps.

PAPER WRAPS   Paper wraps are economical and easy to apply. They are used mainly to repair or patch split or broken nails. Paper wraps are not very strong and are sometimes bulky. Also, they are very visible so polish must be used at all times.

SILK WRAPS   Silk wraps are sheer, very thin (because the weave is tight), and can be worn without polish. The wrap is invisible when applied correctly. Silk wraps are stronger than paper wraps but not as strong as linen or fiberglass. Silk is a truly superior nail fabric material. It is easier to learn than acrylic and requires less filing. **Hint**: Always trim the silk very accurately to the shape of the nail plate and never permit the glue to get into the cuticle area.

If lifting occurs with silk, it is usually caused by using a fabric type of silk, which absorbs too much glue. Always use fine professional type silk. If the silk frays at the cuticle it is usually caused by the client using too much polish remover, which has dissolved the glue holding the silk to the nail.

LINEN WRAPS   Linen wraps are stronger than paper, silk, and fiberglass, and are excellent for treating weak or damaged nails. The wrap is not invisible so polish must be worn. Linen is a thicker wrap than silk because the weave is looser.

FIBERGLASS WRAPS   Fiberglass wraps are the latest of the wrapping services. They combine several of the best qualities of silk and linen wraps. Fiberglass, or "glass" as some refer to it, is a mesh that is thin but has great strength, is transparent, and allows the customer to wear nails natural or polished. The nails are natural looking and feeling.   The wrap is a flexible overlay that, when used properly, will allow the nails to grow out strong and healthy.

The fiberglass system doesn't use primer, liquids, powders, or brushes. It is applied by placing a nail-size piece of fiberglass onto the nail or nail tip and then sealing it in place with an adhesive. It is healthy for natural nails because primer is not used and heavy filing is not necessary. It requires approximately one-tenth as much filing as acrylics. Compared to acrylic, fiberglass wraps are thinner, lighter, nondehydrating, nonporous, odorless, nonyellowing, and stronger. Also, the time required to apply fiberglass is approximately two-thirds that of acrylic sets. Be sure to select a product that is readily available and that has adequate manufacturer support and educational programs.

SCULPTURED NAILS

Many people simply cannot grow long, attractive natural nails. Even those who can will occasionally break a nail and need a replacement or repair quickly. Artificial acrylic nails are strong, durable, natural looking, and easy to polish. Also, they can be worn naturally, without polish, if desired. They look great with a French manicure. With training and practice, full sets of acrylic nails can be applied within two hours.

The acrylic system consists of a polymer (powder) and a monomer (liquid). When the two are combined they create polymerization, a chemical reaction that alters the chemical composition of the two ingredients. The result is a crystallization. Chemically, the result is very similar to Plexiglas™.

Sculptured (acrylic) nails do not harm the natural nails if the proper procedures are followed and with adequate customer nail maintenance. Proper maintenance (fills/repair) is required at least every two weeks. With a longer time period between appointments problems could occur and mold or fungus could develop.

Problems

The problems with acrylic nails are relatively minor. The artificial nails are not flexible so if the nail is hit a hard blow, the natural nail layers could be removed or damaged or damage to the nail plate itself could occur. To be removed, the artificial nails must be soaked off. However, I have worn acrylic nails constantly for years without ever having anything approaching a problem occur.

CHEMICALS   Because of the chemicals, there are vapors that might be uncomfortable or irritating to some individuals. Therefore, adequate salon and workstation ventilation is a must in order to avoid inhaling the chemical vapors and the dust resulting from filing.

Be sure to receive, and retain on file, the full chemical data (MSDS) from the product manufacturer you use. The manufacturer should also be willing and able to answer any questions you may have about the product and its application. If you encounter any form of nonassistance, change the product and the manufacturer.

LIFTING   The biggest problem to guard against with using acrylics is with lifting. Lifting can be caused by many situations. Medical drugs can stay in an individual's system for up to three weeks. Vitamin B6 (a natural diuretic), other diuretics, diet pills, and amphetamines take moisture out of a person's system. Other drugs such as cocaine, thyroid pills, estrogen, and antibiotics change a person's metabolism and can result in lifting of the acrylic nails. Also, natural oils, moisture, a diseased nail plate, excess dirt, nervous habits, occupational hazards, and misuse of tools can also cause lifting to occur. This is why it is so important to have an in depth up-front consultation with every new customer to review in detail their medical history and lifestyle.

PEDICURES

If I were to provide only one service other than nails it would be pedicures. Fees for the service range from $25 to $50, depending on the location of your salon and the type of pedicures you offer. As a first step, check with your local state board for any restrictions on providing the service or on any limitations regarding the use of implements. Some states do not allow beauty or nail salons to provide pedicures.

More women and men are learning to appreciate the benefit of a relaxing and beautifying pedicure, a unique way to be pampered. Pedicures usually take an hour to do and many people like to have them every four to five weeks. A good pedicure is such an exceptional experience that for some it may be a necessary indulgence— once. After that, it's a pure necessity.

You will need to know when it is safe, and when it is not safe to do a pedicure. You must know when to refer a customer to a podiatrist or physician for medical treatment. This will require a consultation with the customer to identify any existing medical conditions or problems. As with other services complete a customer information card with all pertinent information. Never, under any circumstances, attempt to diagnose what is medically "wrong" with a client. This will in essence be practicing medicine without a license.

Your objective in providing pedicures is to provide cosmetic treatment to the client—to beautify the feet, shape and polish the toenails, reduce calluses, massage the feet and the lower legs.

As with other services, a dedicated, specially designed section of the salon should be reserved for pedicures. You can spend anywhere from $50 to $3,000 on a pedicure station. You have to decide whether you are going to start slow and modest or go full-scale ahead with a first class operation. Either way has its advantages and disadvantages.

In addition to realizing income from providing pedicure services, you can generate income from the retailing of home care maintenance products, such as pumice stones, polish, polish remover, top coat, antiseptic spray, and moisturizing lotion. These sales can add an additional 30 to 50 percent of the profits realized from the pedicure services offered.

Safety

Safety is always a major concern with any procedure or service, and pedicures are no exception.

PERIPHERAL VASCULAR DISEASE   Cutting can be dangerous, particularly with peripheral vascular disease, such as arteriosclerosis (hardening of the arteries), because some clients could be on a blood-thinning drug. If you cut someone who has thin blood, sometimes it is difficult to stop the bleeding.

DIABETES   For diabetics, the problem is even more serious. Diabetes is a disorder of carbohydrate metabolism caused by inadequate production or utilization of insulin. Blood circulation is adversely affected, especially in the smaller blood vessels. Sometimes there is a lack of sensation at the end extremities (the feet and hands). Someone with diabetes may not even feel a cut on the foot. Diabetics with poor circulation also tend to get more infections, which they sometimes do not feel. Very severe injury can occur, including gangrene. Many people feel service to diabetics should be limited to massages and the shaping of the toe nails (with a file only), avoiding the use of any cutting instruments.

VARICOSE VEINS   Varicose veins is another problem condition. Veins are like canals with valves that control the blood supply by opening and closing. When these valves cease to function properly the blood tends to "pool" in the veins, resulting in what is called varicose veins. Massage is generally a safe procedure but care must be taken not to injure a vein. Use common sense; avoid working on or around serious looking varicose veins.

CIRCULATORY PROBLEMS   Older clients are more prone to have circulatory problems, which means the feet will be more susceptible to infection because they are farthest from the heart. The feet are also the most difficult place on which to treat and cure an infection because medication does not get to the problem area as easily or as quickly as to other areas of the body.

I would recommend you establish a professional relationship with a local podiatrist. Give the customer the doctor's business card and recommend they come back to you when a condition is corrected.

PARAFFIN (WAX)

Paraffin (wax) was first used by doctors as a therapeutic treatment. It works by trapping heat and moisture in and opening up pores in the skin. The heat from the warm paraffin increases the blood supply to the skin, giving skin that was rough and dry a fresh, soft, healthy feeling. The results are outstanding, so this is a great additional source of income for the salon.

Paraffin is a petroleum by-product that has excellent heat sealing properties. Special units are utilized to melt solid wax into a liquid that is then maintained at a temperature generally between 125 and 130 degrees Fahrenheit. Be sure to follow instructions for whichever unit you may use. Also, if you do provide this service, (which I strongly recommend) use equipment that is designed especially for this treatment. Do not try to heat wax in anything other than the right equipment.

Paraffin treatments are ideal for the hands and feet. Estheticians also use paraffin in their facial treatments (this takes special training and should not be tried by just anyone). The treatments are especially beneficial for senior citizens and people with arthritis. However, anyone can enjoy and benefit from a foot and/or hand paraffin treatment.

Read and follow all operating instructions. Generally you should avoid giving paraffin treatments to anyone who has impaired circulation or skin irritations such as cuts, burns, rashes, warts, eczema, or swollen veins.

If proper procedures are followed, paraffin will not affect artificial nails, wraps, tips, gels, or natural nails. Just make sure all nail repair work is completed before the paraffin treatment, not after.

Paraffin treatments are very easy to provide and require minimum training for the staff. The cost of each treatment to the salon is probably less than $1 for the electricity and wax. Income can range from $5 to $15 depending on the type of clientele you have. Paraffin is an excellent way to pamper your clients and is a profitable service. I just love it.

WAXING

Nail care is the largest growing segment of the beauty industry. Close behind are auxiliary services that are providing additional income and profits. Waxing (hair removal) is one of these services.

Nails and hair removal (epilation) are very compatible services. Every nail customer is a potential client for waxing, (which is quick and relatively uncomplicated) as every woman must have her eyebrows properly shaped and maintained on a monthly basis. Waxing is relatively easy to learn with minimal training. It provides a higher profit margin than nail salon services, if you figure what you make on nail services versus waxing for the same time spent on each service.

Waxing is a relatively quick service with long-lasting results. It is a good repeat service. Waxing done skillfully causes very little pain and is a much better method of hair removal than shaving. With waxing, the hair takes longer to grow back because the wax penetrates into the pore and pulls out the entire hair from the root, or papilla. When a hair is removed by waxing, a new hair must be produced from the follicle, which can take an average of three to six weeks. With repeat treatments the new hair grows out finer and softer.

AVERAGE WAXING SERVICE		
	SERVICE TIME	PRICE
Full leg	45 minutes	$30–40
Arm	20 minutes	20–25
Bikini line	20 minutes	12–15
Eyebrow	15 minutes	7–12
Fingers	10 minutes	5–8
Upper lip	10 minutes	5–8

Be sure to follow the instructions with the particular system you use. Also, be sure to check with your state board to verify the licensing requirements required to provide this service.

SKIN CARE

Skin care is another service you can offer your clients that is a good source of additional income to the salon. And it is another service that keeps your clients coming back to your salon. Women want to look their very best and realize that they will have to invest some time and money to achieve their good looks. You might as well be the provider of that service and get them into your salon as potential customers for your other services. Why should your services end with nails? Beauty aids are a multibillion dollar industry and there is room for you to get a share of the market.

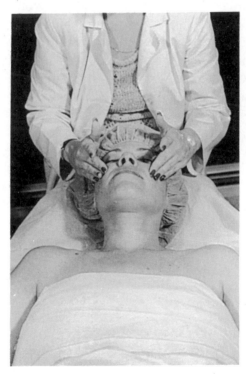

Skin care is another service you can offer your clients that is a good source of additional income to the salon. (Photo courtesy of *Modern Esthetics* by Henry Gambino.)

The skin is the body's largest and most visible organ. There are four basic skin types:

1. Normal skin, which is smooth and moist but not shiny, with pores that are barely visible.
2. Dry skin, which is usually thinner and has less surface oil.
3. Oily skin, which is thick and shiny, due to more oil, and has large noticeable pores.
4. Combination skin, which is normal or dry in most areas but oily on the nose, chin, and forehead.

You will want to merchandise skin care services and products correctly so as to maximize your profit potential. You must have an area dedicated to and specially designed for makeup consultations. Products should be effectively displayed so that they are attractive and inviting, and be sure the client can access them easily. Keep the entire area very clean and neat at all times. Your display shelves must be fully stocked to advertise how successful and confident you are with this service. And always have a makeup artist at your cosmetic counter to invite inquiries and demonstrate your commitment to this service.

If you do not want to manage and be responsible for this service, you might consider renting a space to a makeup artist. This could be a great opportunity for someone starting out and relatively inexpensive compared to having to open her own salon. The price would depend on how much space you provide, what equipment you provide, and by the number of clients you have in your salon. Remember, everything is negotiable.

Skin care is both a science and an art that requires a quiet and relaxing sitting, not only for the treatment but for the initial consultation. The space required could be as little as 100 square feet (10' X 10'). The area should be first class and for the proper facial room the cost will probably be around $3,500.

Make sure the manufacturer you choose has a good educational program and products your clientele desire. Also, make sure your esthetician likes the products and can aggressively sell them.

When selecting an esthetician, you will want one who is not just licensed but is really qualified to give good skin care services. The individual must be fully versed in all aspects of professional treatments and have good customer and interpersonal skills. Last, but certainly not least, this person should be enthusiastic and a self-promoter.

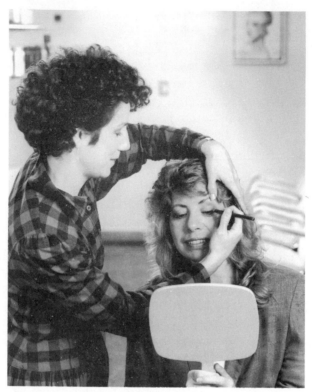

You might consider renting a space to a makeup artist to provide another service for your clients.

MASSAGE

Massage is an old art that can transform a manicure or pedicure into something very special. This is something extra that your salon should provide in your list of services. Study the techniques of the Swedish massage, reflexology, shiatsu, and acupressure. You might want to pick and choose from each to create your own program for use in your salon.

Shiatsu and Acupressure

Shiatsu and acupressure are oriental techniques. People who use these techniques believe that the body's vital energy must be kept free flowing as it passes through the body's major pathways or meridians.

choose to stock a large selection, you will have to order each nail individually. For this you will need a ring of "sizing" nails so as to order the right size for the customer. Depending on the quality, gold nails can be expensive but are very profitable for you. Be sure to receive a sizeable deposit from the customer before you order the nail.

Three-dimensional (3-D) Artwork

Three dimensional (3-D) artwork is one of the latest forms of nail art on the market. This really takes some training or practice and time to do. Again, the designs are all individual and unique. Sculpturing product, various wires, stones, and plastics are used to create designs.

Airbrushing

Airbrushing is a popular form of nail art made by utilizing an airbrush that sprays a very fine paint mist to create a design. Airbrushing can be a substitute for polished nails.

Embossing

Embossing is simply a method of drawing a design on a nail with acrylic paint using a syringelike applicator. Each design is unique to what the customer wants. It is a method of creating raised dots, lines, and commas to form countless patterns on the customer's nails. It has been described as painting-by-the-numbers. No experience is required. The manufacturer provides detailed, step-by-step instructions that don't require talent. An embossing tool is used to create the patterns and is very easy to use. The paint used is a thick, water-based acrylic, which is malleable and doesn't shrink when it dries. It is almost like decorating pastry.

The cost to start this service is relatively low. You can get a starter kit with six basic colors, accompanying tool, and instruction book for under $50. Designs are limited only by your imagination. The profit potential to your salon is excellent.

COLOR ANALYSIS

Color analysis is another service you may want to consider. I have found that color analysis specialists are always amazing. People who think they have an eye for color are usually surprised to find out which colors complement them the best. You can find color analysis courses that last anywhere from two weeks to two years. Check out the ones in your area very carefully before you invest your money. If this service is not readily available elsewhere, you might want to consider providing it.

EAR PIERCING

This should also be considered as a service to provide to your customers. While you obviously will not have many repeat customers, the service is still a profitable one. Be sure the system you choose meets the Food and Drug Administration (FDA) standards and that you provide adequate training to whoever performs this service.

You might want to consider an arrangement whereby you have someone come in one day a week to provide this service. You could maintain an appointment book and work out how you would split the income. This way you wouldn't have any investment to make but would still be providing a service and generating additional income for the salon.

SPECIAL SERVICES

Services to shut-ins, nursing homes, retirement homes, and luxury hotels may be appropriate in your area. First, however, for anything you do out of the ordinary be sure to check with the regulatory agency in your state. Be sure what you want to do will be allowed. Special services may also include pedicures for expectant mothers and/or new mothers and for professionals with hectic schedules. Luxury hotel room services may be an option for guests who are too ill to travel or guests who are too well known and want to guard their privacy.

In addition to all of the above, and again depending on your finances, the availability of qualified employees, the location of your salon, the demographics of your clientele, your available salon space, and your competition, you might want to consider other product lines to offer, such as lingerie, cruise and beachwear, evening wear, jewelry, and wigs.

If you do get involved with additional products and services you might consider organizing your own fashion and beauty shows for men and women to show off all your services and retail items. This could become a fun and profitable event for your salon, staff, and customers.

NAIL POLISH

You must have a large supply of nail polish in a wide variety of colors. However, don't overstock. You should keep a three-to-six-month supply in stock at all times. The shelf life of nail polish is two years, but ideally it should be used within a year of bottling.

Store nail polish at below seventy degrees Fahrenheit. If nail polish is exposed to sunlight it could expand and explode. If it thickens, thin with a drop of thinner (never thin with polish remover).

Nail polishing is an art that may require a lot of practice to perfect. Even though some people have a difficult time learning to polish well, it can be learned. Three steady strokes should completely cover a nail.

Polish bubbling occurs when you don't allow sufficient drying time between coats of polish and/or you shake the polish bottle and create air bubbles. For polish to dry the solvents in the nail polish must dissipate. There are three major components of nail polish (butylacetate, toluene, and nitrocellulose) that must dry in a predetermined order for ideal results. Too much cold or too much heat will alter the drying cycle.

Nail polish should be dried at between seventy and ninety-five degrees Fahrenheit. Be sure to allow adequate time, at least thirty seconds, between layers of polish to prevent streaking, bubbling, and uneven drying. Each coat of polish will dry at a different rate. **Note:** nails must be completely dry and free of oil prior to polishing.

PRODUCT SALES

You can increase your salon profits significantly by selling retail items. Make available to your customers the products they need and use that they would otherwise purchase somewhere else. Start retailing the everyday supplies like glue, polish, polish remover, and files; items that your clients need to maintain their nails. Simply increase your normal purchases of these products gradually as you start your retailing program. Avoid introducing a variety of items at once. Focus on a few items at a time and build up gradually. Then reinvest your profits in additional products.

Product Line

As you expand your product line, offer only items that appeal to your clients, not to the general public. By offering convenience and personalized service you will be able to convert salon space into a profit center.

Avoid competing with large department stores. Don't offer the same items that could be purchased elsewhere at a lower price because of their volume discount purchasing. Also, avoid "trendy" items that can leave you with unsold inventory that can go out of style very quickly. This gets very expensive, especially for a small retail operation that cannot absorb the loss.

A successful salon retail program requires a combination of the right products, right price, and right style. This will result in additional profit for the salon. Don't miss out on this opportunity.

Your product line should be based on the make up of your clientele, their income levels, their needs, and what they like to buy. Your product line should be as exclusive as possible so as to retain its appeal. You will want to emphasize quality and style.

Be sure to price your products clearly and correctly, not too high or too low. Be imaginative and creative with your product display, making it attractive, inviting and convenient for the customer, preferably in or near the reception area. Remember to keep the display area clean and neat at all times. All employees, both technicians and the receptionist, should be actively involved with retail sales.

Provide sales training as part of your education schedule. Try to bring in outside specialists to help educate your staff and keep enthusiasm high.

Try to attend at least one or two trade shows a year, especially the larger ones. This is a good way to stay abreast of what is new and provides an excellent opportunity to discuss any issues or concerns with the product manufacturer representative. Many manufacturers have show specials for their products that can save you money. Also, most have demonstrations of their products at the trade shows.

Be careful not to shop for price only. Your customers are coming to you for special "professional" treatment—that means the best available. My own experience confirms that people are willing to pay for quality. However, no one is willing to pay premium prices for poor quality products, or service.

Be aware that all products will not work on all people. You may require different product lines to accommodate your individual clients.

Once you become comfortable with a product try to order it in bulk quantities. This way you save time and money.

Before we get off products, if you don't already know how, learn to read labels. Ingredients are listed in order of quantity—the largest volume ingredient is listed first, the second largest by volume is listed second, etc. Be aware of perfumes added to lotions. Note the ingredients and be sure a client is not allergic to any of them.

Private Label Products

Private label products are growing in popularity and may be something you should consider. Private label is simply the practice of selling products that carry your salon's name. This is not something you should consider lightly, however, because you are associating your salon name and reputation to the product.

Usually, private label cosmetic costs are less expensive than brand name cosmetics thus resulting in a higher profit margin. Since the salon label/logo is on each item additional salon exposure is achieved. Also, your salon will be the only source for the particular item or brand. But since it is a private label item, the salon is responsible for the promotion and creation of buyer interest since there will not be any large advertising campaign behind it as with national brand names. You must give as much thought and planning to this venture as you did to the decor, physical location, and style of the salon itself.

The product or item (usually cosmetics) must be of a quality to stand up to discriminating customers, otherwise the salon's reputation and level of business will suffer.

In deciding whether to pursue this idea you must first evaluate the potential profitability of the items. You must also evaluate whether your clientele will accept the products, your own marketing skills, and your staff's level of commitment. Just as important is deciding whether you have the time, commitment, and ability to sell private label products.

If you decide to proceed beyond this point, you will have to find a source for your supply, either a manufacturer, wholesaler or distributor. You will need to evaluate the quality of what is available and what assistance different companies offer (sales, technical, marketing, packaging). In addition you will need to evaluate shipping costs, payment policies, quantity requirements, and quality for each potential source. Determine if incentives are available, such as discounts, promotion, literature, or displays.

Then you must consider design and packaging. The supplier may be able to help with this or you may need to go to a separate packaging designer. You will probably have to choose between a traditional label or silk screening, which will be decided by your budget and the image you wish to convey to your clientele. Then you will have to design the label and decide what you want on it (in addition to your salon name and phone number).

You may want to start small (as with nail polish) and gradually add other items depending on your personal inclination, the success of the initial phase, and the perceived difficulties to be faced. This is an involved decision but if you decide to proceed do so with the knowledge that it will take planning, research, work, and a sustained commitment to be successful.

PRICING

Establishing the prices for your services begins with analyzing many factors, including the type, location, and skill of your salon staff; community demographics; and your competition.

Skill Level

Sometimes it is difficult to be realistic about our own skill levels. But some key indicators would be:

- Comments from customers regarding your staff and operations.
- The extent/quality of your expertise and staff planning.
- Whether you have long-term customers or a high customer turnover.
- Whether your customers refer their friends to your salon.
- Do you provide a full range of services or do you need to train in the areas of services you don't provide?

Community Demographics

Also consider what type of community you are located in. Are you in an expensive, upper income area that is style conscious, with women who don't work or a working-class, blue-collar area with high unemployment? Or are you somewhere in between?

Competition

You also must consider your competition. Try to identify three or four competitors with services similar to your salon's and check their prices. Simply average the individual totals and you have a starting point on which to base your price.

Pricing Levels

You might also want to consider several pricing levels for some of your services instead of a single charge. For example a basic manicure treatment, a regular manicure, and a deluxe manicure would each have its own price level.

You might also have a price level by technician if there are significant differences in their skill levels. This would be particularly appropriate with new, relatively inexperienced employees just starting to build up their own clientele base.

Price Increases

You will need to constantly be sensitive to this price issue and to the question of when you should increase your prices. You will need to raise your pricing when/if:

1. Your costs increase (inventory, rent, salaries, utilities, insurance, taxes, etc.).
2. To remain competitive. (You don't want to be the lowest price in your community if other salons can charge more for similar services.)
3. You do an extensive remodeling.
4. You want to reduce your clientele to a smaller, select few, who will accept higher pricing.

If you do find it necessary to increase your pricing, be sure to give your customers plenty of notice, both verbally and in writing by posting your price changes. This is only ethical and will protect you legally. Encourage the receptionist and technicians to make sure everyone is informed of the increase. Also, don't consider raising your prices if you are not fully booked and have a waiting list. Once you are fully booked you then can justify increasing prices for your services.

Customers will pay for superior service, even if it costs more. With superior service you do not have to compete with price.

Pricing Products

Pricing products for retail sale is relatively simple. Start with the cost of the item, double it, then add the shipping and handling cost. If you pay any commission to your staff for product sales, add this in also. Then add an amount for advertising if you run a promotion for this particular item.

Another tip is to price each item on its bottom to encourage the customer to pick it up for closer review. This helps to sell the product.

SUMMARY

The services and products you offer in your salon are the reason your customers come to you. Be sure to provide quality in every service you offer and every product you sell. Your prices should reflect that quality and be based on the skill of your salon, your demographics, and your competition.

The more services you offer, the better your salon will be. Manicures, pedicures, and nail care are all important, but do not overlook other possibilities. Waxing, skin care, and massage all fit into a nail salon and can all be very profitable. Related areas, such as color analysis and ear piercing, can be assets to your salon as well.

Product sales can add significant income to your salon. Just be sure that what you offer cannot be purchased at a lower price elsewhere and meets your standards of quality. You may also want to consider private label products, but again be certain of the quality—your salon name and reputation are at stake.

ASSOCIATIONS

A P P E N D I X

A

ALLIED BEAUTY ASSOCIATION
2 Sheppard Ave., E., Suite 1001
Box 42
Villowdale, Ontario M2N 5Y7 Canada
(416) 225-2359

AMERICAN BEAUTY ASSOCIATION
401 North Michigan Ave.
Chicago, IL 60611
(312) 644-6610

AMERICAN WOMAN'S ECONOMIC
DEVELOPMENT CORPORATION
71 Vanderbilt Ave., Suite 320
New York, NY 10169
(212) 692-9100

ASSOCIATION OF ACCREDITED
COSMETOLOGY SCHOOLS
Teachers' Educational Council
(TEC/AACS)
5201 Leesburg Pike, Suite 205
Falls Church, VA 22041
(703) 845-1333

ASSOCIATION OF BRIDAL
CONSULTANTS
200 Chestnutland Rd.
New Milford, CT 06776
(203) 355-0464

ASSOCIATION OF COSMETOLOGISTS
AND HAIRDRESSERS
1811 Monroe
Dearborn, MI 48124
(313) 563-0360

COSMETIC EXECUTIVE WOMEN
217 East 85th St., Suite 214
New York, NY 10028
(212) 535-6117

THE COSMETIC, TOILETRY AND
FRAGRANCE ASSOCIATION
1101 17th St., Suite 300
Washington, DC 20036
(202) 331-1770

ESTHETICIANS INTERNATIONAL
ASSOCIATION
4447 McKinney Ave.
Dallas, Texas 75205
(214) 526-0752

FOOD AND DRUG ADMINISTRATION
5600 Fishers Ln.
Rockville, MD 20857
(301) 295-8063

INTERNATIONAL CHAIN SALON
ASSOCIATION
2440 West 12th Ave.
Vancouver, BC V6K 2N2 Canada
(604) 738-3135

INTERNATIONAL INSTITUTE OF
REFLEXOLOGY
P.O. Box 12642
St. Petersburg, FL 33733-2642

INTERNATIONAL NAIL & BEAUTY
ASSOCIATION
457 Busse Rd.
Elk Grove Village, IL 60007
(708) 956-1040

THE NAIL MANUFACTURERS
COUNCIL
c/o ABA
401 North Michigan Ave.
Chicago, IL 60611
(312) 644-6610

NAIL TECHNICIANS OF AMERICA
c/o NCA
3510 Olive St.
St. Louis, MO 63103
(314) 534-7980

NATIONAL ASSOCIATION OF BLACK
WOMEN'S ENTREPRENEURS
P.O.Box 1375
Detroit, MI 48231
(313) 341-7400

NATIONAL ASSOCIATION OF
FEMALE EXECUTIVES
127 West 24th St.
New York, NY 10011
(212) 645-0770

NATIONAL ASSOCIATION OF STATE
DEVELOPMENT AGENCIES
444 N. Capitol St.
Washington, DC 20001
(202) 898-1302

NATIONAL ASSOCIATION OF
WOMEN BUSINESS OWNERS
600 South Federal St., Suite 400
Chicago, IL 60605
(312) 922-0465

NATIONAL BEAUTY CULTURISTS'
LEAGUE
25 Logan Circle N.W.
Washington, DC 20005
(202) 332-2695

NATIONAL-INTERSTATE COUNCIL
OF STATE BOARDS OF
COSMETOLOGY
1301 Gervais St.
17th Floor-NCNB Tower
P.O. Box 11390
Columbia, SC 29201
(803) 799-9800

NEWSLETTER PUBLISHING
ASSOCIATION
1401 Wilson Blvd., Suite 403
Arlington, VA 22209
(703) 527-2333

OFFICE OF WOMEN'S BUSINESS
OWNERSHIP
U.S. Small Business Administration
1441 L St., N.W., Room 414
Washington, DC 20416

SMALL BUSINESS ADMINISTRATION
P.O. Box 1000
Fort Worth, TX 76119
800-827-5722

WORLD INTERNATIONAL NAIL AND
BEAUTY ASSOCIATION (WINBA)
1221 N. Lakeview
Anaheim, CA 92807
(714) 779-9883

INDIVIDUAL STATE OFFICES FOR DEVELOPMENTAL ASSISTANCE

A P P E N D I X

B

ALABAMA
Alabama Development Office
State Capitol
Montgomery, AL 36130
(800) 248-0033
(205) 263-0048

ALASKA
Division of Economic Development
Department of Commerce and
Economic Development
P.O.Box D
Juneau, AL 99811
(907) 465-2017

ARIZONA
Office of Business Finance
Department of Commerce
3800 North Central Ave., Suite 1500
Phoenix, AZ 85012
(602) 682-5275

ARKANSAS
Small Business Information Center
Industrial Development Commission
State Capitol Mall
Room 4C-300
Little Rock, AR 72201
(501) 682-5275

CALIFORNIA
Office of Small Business
Department of Commerce
801 K St., Suite 1700
Sacramento, CA 95814
(916) 327-4357 (916) 445-6545

COLORADO
One-Stop Assistance Center
1560 Broadway, Suite 1530
Denver, CO 80202
(800) 333-7798 (303) 592-5920

CONNECTICUT
Small Business Services
Department of Economic Development
865 Brook St.
Rocky Hill, CT 06067
(203) 258-4269

DELAWARE
Development Office
P.O. Box 1401
99 Kings Highway
Dover, DE 19903
(302) 739-4271

DISTRICT OF COLUMBIA
Office of Business and
Economic Development
Tenth Floor
717 14th St. N.W.
Washington, DC 20005
(202) 727-6600

FLORIDA
Bureau of Business Assistance
Department of Commerce
107 West Gains St., Room 443
Tallahassee, FL 32399-2000
(800) 342-0771 (904) 488-9357

GEORGIA
Department of Community Affairs
100 Peachtree St., Suite 1200
Atlanta, Ga. 30303
(404) 656-6200

HAWAII
Small Business Information Service
737 Bishop St., Suite 1900
Honolulu, HI 86813
(808) 548-7645 (808) 543-6691

IDAHO
Economic Development Division
Department of Commerce
700 State St.
Boise, ID 83720-2700
(208) 334-2470

ILLINOIS
Small Business Assistance Bureau
Department of Commerce
Community Affairs
620 East Adams St.
Springfield, IL 62701
(800) 252-2923

INDIANA
Ombudsman's Office
Business Development Division
Department of Commerce
One North Capitol, Suite 700
Indianapolis, IN 46204-2288
(800) 824-2476 (317) 232-7304

IOWA
Bureau of Small Business Development
Department of Economic Development
200 East Grand Ave.
Des Moines, IA 50309
(800) 532-1216 (515) 242-4899

KANSAS
Division of Existing Industry
Development
400 SW Eight St.
Topeka, KS 66603
(913) 296-5298

KENTUCKY
Division of Small Business
Capitol Plaza Tower
Frankfort, KY 40601
(800) 626-2250

LOUISIANA
Development Division
Office of Commerce and Industry
P.O. Box 94185
Baton Rouge, LA 70804-9185
(504) 342-5365

MAINE
Business Development Division
State Development Office
State House
Augusta, ME 04333
(800) 872-3838 (207) 289-3153

MARYLAND
Division of Business Development
Department of Economic and
Employment Development
217 East Redwood St.
Baltimore, MD 21202
(800) 873-7232 (301) 333-6996

MASSACHUSETTS
Office of Business Development
100 Cambridge St., 13th Floor
Boston, MA 02202
(617) 727-3206

MICHIGAN
Michigan Business Ombudsman
Department of Commerce
P.O. Box 30107
Lansing, MI 48909
(800) 232-2727 (517) 373-6241

MINNESOTA
Small Business Assistance Office
Department of Trade and
Economic Development
900 American Center Bldg.
150 East Kellogg Blvd.
St. Paul, MN 55101
(800) 652-9747 (612) 296-3871

MISSISSIPPI
Small Business Bureau
Research and Development Center
P.O. Box 849
Jackson, MS 39205
(601) 359-3552

MISSOURI
Small Business Development Office
Department of Economic Development
P.O. Box 118
Jefferson City, MO 65102
(314) 751-4982

MONTANA
Business Assistance Division
Department of Commerce
1424 Ninth Ave.
Helena, MT 59620
(800) 221-8015 (406) 444-2801

NEBRASKA
Existing Business Division
Department of Economic Development
P.O. Box 94666
301 Centennial Mall South
Lincoln, NE 68509-4666
(402) 471-3782

NEVADA
Nevada Commission on Economic
Development
Capitol Complex
Carson City, NV 89710
(702) 687-4325

NEW HAMPSHIRE
Small Business Development Center
University Center, Room 311
400 Commercial St.
Manchester, NH 03101
(603) 625-4522

NEW JERSEY
Office of Small Business Assistance
Department of Commerce and Economic
Development
20 West State St., Cn 835
Trenton, NJ 08625
(609) 984-4442

NEW MEXICO
Economic Development Division
Department of Economic Development
1100 St. Francis Dr.
Santa Fe, NM 87503
(505) 827-0300

NEW YORK
Division For Small Business
Department of Economic Development
1515 Broadway, 51st Floor
New York, NY 10036
(212) 827-6150

NORTH CAROLINA
Small Business Development Division
Department of Economic and
Community Development
Dobbs Bldg., Room 2019
430 North Salisbury St.
Raleigh, NC 27611
(919) 733-7980

NORTH DAKOTA
Small Business Coordinator
Economic Development Commission
Liberty Memorial Building
604 East Blvd.
Bismark, ND 58505
(701) 224-2810

OHIO
Small and Developing Business Division
Department of Development
P.O. Box 1001
Columbus, OH 43266-0101
(800) 248-4040 (614) 466-4232

OKLAHOMA
Oklahoma Department of Commerce
P.O. Box 26980
6601 N. Broadway Extension
Oklahoma City, OK 73126-0980
(800) 477-6552 (405) 843-9770

OREGON
Economic Development Department
775 Summer St. NE
Salem, OR 97310
(800) 233-3306 (503) 373-1200

PENNSYLVANIA
Bureau of Small Business and
Appalachian Development
Department of Commerce
461 Forum Building
Harrisburg, PA 17120
(717) 783-5700

PUERTO RICO
Commonwealth Department of
Commerce
Bos S
4275 Old San Juan Station
San Juan, PR 00905
(809) 721-3290

RHODE ISLAND
Business Development Division
Department of Economic Development
Seven Jackson Walkway
Providence, RI 02903
(401) 277-2601

SOUTH CAROLINA
Enterprise Development
P.O. Box 1149
Columbia, SC 29202
(800) 922-6684 (803) 737-0888

SOUTH DAKOTA
Governor's Office of Economic
Development
Capitol Lake Plaza
711 Wells Ave.
Pierre, SD 57501
(800) 872-6190 (605) 773-5032

TENNESSEE
Small Business Office
Department of Economic and
Community Development
320 Sixth Ave. North
Seventh Floor
Rachel Jackson Building
Nashville, TN 37219
(800) 872-7201 (615) 741-2626

TEXAS
Small Business Division
Department of Commerce
Economic Development Commission
P.O. Box 12728
Capitol Station
410 East Fifth St.
Austin, TX 78711
(800) 888-0511 (512) 472-5059

UTAH
Small Business Development Center
102 West 500 South
Suite 315
Salt Lake City, UT 84101
(801) 581-7905

VERMONT
Agency of Development and
Community Affairs
The Pavillion
109 State St.
Montpelier, VT 05609
(800) 622-4553 (802) 828-3221

VIRGINIA
Small Business and Financial Services
Department of Economic Development
P.O. Box 798
1000 Washington Building
Richmond, VA 23206
(804) 371-8252

WASHINGTON
Small Business Development Center
245 Todd Hall
Washington State University
Pullman, WA 99164-4727
(509) 335-1576

WEST VIRGINIA
Small Business Development Center
Division
1115 Virginia St. East
Charleston, WV 25301
(304) 348-2960

WISCONSIN
Public Information Bureau
Department of Development
P.O. Box 7970
123 West Washington Ave.
Madison, WI 53707
(800) 435-7287 (608) 266-1018

WYOMING
Economic Development and
Stabilization Board
Herschler Building
Cheyenne, WY 82002
(307) 777-7287

STATE BOARDS OF COSMETOLOGY

A P P E N D I X

C

ALABAMA	(205) 261-5613	MONTANA	(406) 444-4288
ALASKA	(907) 465-2547	NEBRASKA	(402) 471-2115
ARIZONA	(602) 542-5301	NEVADA	(702) 486-6542
ARKANSAS	(501) 682-2168	NEW HAMPSHIRE	(603) 271-3608
CALIFORNIA	(916) 445-7061	NEW JERSEY	(201) 504-6400
COLORADO	(303) 894-7772	NEW MEXICO	(505) 827-7176
CONNECTICUT	(203) 566-4068	NEW YORK	(212) 587-5747
DELAWARE	(302) 739-4522	NORTH CAROLINA	(919) 850-2793
FLORIDA	(904) 488-5702	NORTH DAKOTA	(701) 224-9800
GEORGIA	(404) 656-3909	OHIO	(614) 466-3834
HAWAII	(808) 586-2699	OKLAHOMA	(405) 521-2441
IDAHO	(208) 334-3233	OREGON	(503) 378-8667
ILLINOIS	(217) 785-0800	PENNSYLVANIA	(717) 783-7130
INDIANA	(317) 232-2980	RHODE ISLAND	(401) 277-2511
IOWA	(515) 281-4422	SOUTH CAROLINA	(803) 734-9660
KANSAS	(913) 296-3155	SOUTH DAKOTA	(605) 224-5072
KENTUCKY	(502) 564-4262	TENNESSEE	(615) 741-2515
LOUISIANA	(504) 295-8476	TEXAS	(512) 454-4674
MAINE	(207) 582-8745	UTAH	(801) 530-6628
MARYLAND	(410) 333-6320	VERMONT	(802) 828-2373
MASSACHUSETTS	(617) 727-9940	VIRGINIA	(804) 367-3509
MICHIGAN	(517) 373-0580	WASHINGTON	(206) 586-6359
MINNESOTA	(612) 297-7050	WEST VIRGINIA	(304) 558-2924
MISSISSIPPI	(601) 354-6623	WISCONSIN	(608) 266-1630
MISSOURI	(314) 751-1052	WYOMING	(307) 265-2917

INDEX

Note: Page numbers in **bold type** reference non-text material.